INSIDE THE MENTAL

INSIDE
THE MENTAL

SILENCE, STIGMA, PSYCHIATRY, AND LSD

KAY PARLEY

υ?

My own experiences related in *Inside The Mental* are factual, but some of the names and details
concerning other patients and staff at the hospital have been altered to protect their privacy.

Printed and bound in Canada at Friesens.

COVER AND TEXT DESIGN: Duncan Campbell, University of Regina Press
COPY EDITOR: Joan McGilvray   PROOFREADER: Kristine Douaud
COVER PHOTO: Carrie Fijal Kaye / Snapwire

Library and Archives Canada Cataloguing in Publication

Parley, Kay, author

Inside the mental : silence, stigma, psychiatry, and LSD / Kay Parley.

(The Regina collection)

Parts of this work were included in Lady with a lantern.

Issued in print and electronic formats. ISBN 978-0-88977-411-7 (hardback).
—ISBN 978-0-88977-413-1 (html).—ISBN 978-0-88977-412-4 (pdf)

1. Parley, Kay—Health. 2. Weyburn Mental Hospital—History. 3. Psychiatry—
Saskatchewan—History. 4. LSD (Drug)—Therapeutic use—Saskatchewan—
History. 5. Psychiatric nurses—Saskatchewan—Biography. 6. Psychotherapy
patients—Saskatchewan—Biography. I. Title. II. Series: Regina collection

RC448.S33W49 2016   362.2'1097124   C2016-900155-5   C2016-900156-3

University of Regina Press

Saskatchewan, Canada, S4S 0A2
TEL: (306) 585-4758 FAX: (306) 585-4699
WEB: www.uofrpress.ca

10 9 8 7 6 5 4 3 2 1

We acknowledge the support of the Canada Council for the Arts for our publishing
program. We acknowledge the financial support of the Government of Canada. / Nous
reconnaissons l'appui financier du gouvernement du Canada. This publication was made
possible through Creative Saskatchewan's Creative Industries Production Grant Program.

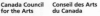
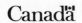

*To anyone and everyone
who fights the stigma*

Kathleen

She was just a half a person,
Six or seven, skinny, meek,
Heart a mass of fissures, brain in prison,
Will is weak;
Flailing at a foreign world,
Eating gall and drinking tears,
Hidden from reality through
Fifty bitter years.
How hard it's been to help her,
She's the saddest thing I've seen—
But it's harder still to realize—admit—
That I'm Kathleen.

From The Multiple Personality Poems *by Kay Parley*

CONTENTS

ACKNOWLEDGEMENTS

The people who contributed indirectly to this book are too numerous to list and, since I am ninety-three, not many will be alive to read their names. But I want to express gratitude to those who helped me through my 1948 breakdown: my mother, who made sure I received treatment, Dr. R. J. Weil, Dr. Z. Selinger, and so many of the staff at the Weyburn mental hospital. Then there are those who eased me—in fact boosted me—through the difficult time of rehabilitation: Larry Lowes, Jean Arnett Freeman, Mavis Jahnke, and N. R. MacDonald. There were many more. I wish I had room to thank all those who offered support and stimulation, enriching my training as a registered psychiatric nurse: especially Dr. Humphrey Osmond, Francis Huxley, and

Dr. Gwyn Gilliland. For the camaraderie I found at University Hospital, thank you to all.

A big thank you to my publisher, Bruce Walsh of University of Regina Press for the sensitivity he has shown in seeing potential value in these stories. Thank you, too, to Joan McGilvray for the great job she did selecting passages from my writing to be included in the book. As for my editor, David McLennan, I can't imagine finding anyone more compatible and understanding. Working with him has been a terrific experience.

To all those who helped me live this story and to those who have done so much to organize and prepare the book, my most sincere thank you.

CREDITS

Much of the material in *Inside The Mental* is compiled from a number of my earlier publications:

"Toppling a Monument" and "Psychiatric Nurse" were first published as part of an article in *The Journal of Orthomolecular Psychiatry* vol. 6, no. 1 (1977): 63–68.

"The Nameless Threats" is excerpted from "Living with Schizophrenia," first published under my pseudonym, Norma MacDonald, in *The Canadian Medical Association Journal* vol. 82 (Jan. 23, 1960): 218-221.

"Psychiatric Patient" is excerpted from "The Lady with the Healing Hands," first published in the magazine of the Canadian Mental Health Association, Saskatchewan Division, *Transition* (Fall 2003): 72–75.

Also first published in *Transition* were "Christmas Comes to The Mental," *Transition* (Winter 1996), 12– 24; "The Torch," *Transition* (Spring 2006), 87–89; and "Night of the Red Rug," *Transition* (Fall 2007), 4–6.

"Meeting Grandpa" was first published in our family history, *Dyer Consequences*, now housed in the Saskatchewan Genealogy library, Regina, Saskatchewan.

"Kleckner" was first published in *Prism International* vol. 5, no. 2 (Autumn 1965).

"LSD" was first published as "LSD—A Backward Glance at the Sixties by One Who Saw the Best of It" in *The Wolseley Bulletin,* November 23, 2012.

"Supporting the Patient on LSD Day" first appeared in *The American Journal of Nursing* (February 1964), 80–82.

"Sunday," "The Glass of Truth," "Understanding," "An Afternoon in the Sun," and "Community" are excerpted from the journal and other material first published in my self-published volume "Lady with a Lantern" (2007).

INTRODUCTION

The stories in this book cover a fairly wide spectrum in time and subject matter, from treatments available in the mental hospital at Weyburn, Saskatchewan, in 1948 to what it was like to do psychiatric nursing in the same hospital during the enlightened fifties, to a peek at the fascinating research being done with LSD in the sixties. Perhaps the unity to be found in the stories is the writer herself, because I had the good fortune to experience all of that.

Mental illness was always part of my life. When I was born, my maternal grandfather, diagnosed as paranoid, was already in the Weyburn hospital, which was commonly called "The Big Mental" or "The Mental." I had never seen my grandfather, so his absence didn't make a difference to me, but when I was only six my father was taken to the same hospital with a diagnosis of manic-depressive psychosis. My world shattered. I'd been a "Daddy's girl," so I lost much of the love in my life at that tender age. I handled it in one of the worst ways possible, by repression. My emotions froze. I remembered almost nothing of the days when Dad had been at home, nothing at all of the anguish I'd endured when I found that he was gone. Forgetting saved me from disintegration, and the fact that my intellectual and creative capacities were unharmed enabled me to carry on fairly normally and to do well in school. Still, emotional instability is destructive. By the time I was twenty-four I'd changed careers four or five times, lost the one serious love of my life, and developed a multiple personality. I never "split," as happens in extreme cases of multiple personality, but one of the girls living in me led me up false paths for years, because she was determined to be an actress and I was neither talented enough nor motivated enough to be a success in drama.

People seldom realized how depressed or confused I could be, so I took a lot of criticism. A psychiatrist once told me I gave people "the wrong signals," so it was my own fault if I was misunderstood. My mother had a very high IQ and held "reason" in high regard, but she had no time for emotion, so I got almost no emotional support. In 1948, while doing office work at CBC Radio in Toronto,

I fell apart. My practical mother whisked me home to Saskatchewan and got me into treatment.

That is when I finally met my father and my grandfather and when I learned what a mental hospital was really like. The first thing my psychiatrist explained was that I had ceased to develop emotionally at the age of seven. I was now twenty-five. I had lost eighteen years, and he told me it would take eighteen years to catch up. It did.

I can't say I loved the mental hospital without misgivings. It was crowded, noisy, smelly, shabby, with too much authority around and too many people who behaved in threatening or in particularly unintelligent ways. But in many ways I loved The Big Mental. It was home to so many people, and some of the "old-timers" were very receptive. We had therapists who were warm, friendly, understanding, and encouraging. After nine months I was discharged from the admitting ward to work in Weyburn. The city was used to mental patients and I was welcomed into a rooming house where I felt right at home. I joined an art class, helped start a little theatre, and felt better than I ever had. I worked in a law office and was doing well, but then the newly formed Saskatchewan Arts Board offered me a job and I thought I should return to Regina. Two years later, in 1954, I was back in Toronto and . . .!!! Another breakdown.

It was so familiar I simply let it happen. I followed the advice my psychiatrists had given me: ate well, got my sleep, took healthy walks, and stayed out of work until I was broke. It took four months. Then I was able to take a job with Office Overload and pull myself back up again. I had no idea what my illness was. They hadn't given me a diagnosis at Weyburn, but I was afraid it might be manic-depressive psychosis, like my Dad. I'd read a bit about it in the mental hospital library and learned that it was cyclic and recurring, but that the episodes were self-curing. I'd get well, with or without therapy.

At that point I'd forgotten about the summer of 1942, the first year I'd had a job. I'd been so upset that my mother took me to a doctor and he told me to "grow up." (That's how much they knew about mental illness in 1942.) Had I remembered that experience, I would have been more worried, because 1942 to 1948 to 1954 indicated six-year intervals. Recurrent at regular intervals. I didn't want to have to face that. But it did enter my mind that perhaps I might be able to work in psychiatry. It looked as if events in my life were pushing me that way. Still, I didn't like the way the hospital was organized well enough to want to be part of its military discipline. Then I got the letter.

A Weyburn friend wrote to tell me there was a new superintendent at the mental hospital with new ideas. He was making a lot of changes. She wrote, "We're hearing good things about the hospital."

Could *I* be a psychiatric nurse? I'd never wanted to be a nurse. I'd trained for commercial art, stenography and radio, and I'd been a country schoolteacher for three years—but nursing? I felt as if destiny was chasing me. My life was too involved with mental illness for me to ignore it. I was concerned about all those people I'd known in the hospital. I'd watched some struggle through rehabilitation, as I had. Two of those friends had already lost the struggle and committed suicide. Could I be of any use?

My Dad had left hospital and built himself a little bungalow by the Souris River, right beside the mental hospital grounds in Weyburn. I decided to return to Saskatchewan and pay him a visit. I ended up spending the winter with Dad. I had been publishing stories for four years, so I did some writing, but it took until March 1956 to get up the courage to walk over to the mental hospital and apply to go on staff.

In the seven years since my discharge, the hospital had moved so far from the place I'd known in the winter of 1948–49 as to be almost unrecognizable. There were crafts and recreational activities going on right on the wards. Remodelling and modernizing was in progress. The grounds were filled with life. The friendlier, more relaxed atmosphere was tangible. Patients with jobs in the hospital had pass keys and could let themselves through the locked doors. There was a healthier, more hopeful feeling in the air.

I began to work at the newly named Saskatchewan Hospital at Weyburn in March, 1956, and graduated as a Registered Psychiatric Nurse in 1959. In 1957 the American Psychiatric Association gave the Weyburn hospital an achievement award as the North American Mental Hospital making the most progress. I felt I'd hit the crest of a wave: Saskatchewan was leading the field and the world was watching.

The research going on was largely biochemical experiments conducted in Saskatoon by the head of research, Dr. Abram Hoffer. I knew very little about those. Our superintendent, Dr. Humphry Osmond, was an enthusiastic partner to Dr. Hoffer, and our research department was doing studies of group interaction and lots on perception. We were also involved with the new experimentation with lysergic acid diethylamide (LSD). The focus was on trying to find the cause of and cure for schizophrenia, the illness that had devastated so many of our patients. The doctors were so focused on this that we sometimes joked that they saw every patient admitted as schizophrenic. I fell under that banner: I had endured numerous auditory hallucinations and perhaps a bit of false visual perception, so my field of perception was considered "fluid," and a fluid perceptual field was the current definition of schizophrenia. Dr. Osmond even asked me to write an article for a medical journal entitled "Living with Schizophrenia." I wrote it, calling on some of my memories of the "down" times of my illness, but I used a pseudonym and hoped it wouldn't get much attention. I still had no diagnosis but I couldn't see much resemblance between myself and the many schizophrenic patients around me. Yet the idea gave me a ray of hope. If it was schizophrenia I had, I had actually conquered it. I'd recovered from two breakdowns. If it wasn't MDP after all, it might not reoccur.

Of course it did. I had breakdowns every six years with clockwork precision and I handled them all with the simple rules my psychiatrists had given me in 1949. I never took medication. My doctor hadn't even given me sleeping pills, believing I had to handle it on my own, with guts. It worked. Until my fifth breakdown in 1972, I never saw a psychiatrist again. That time I was lecturing in social sciences at a technical institute, and trying to lecture with an inner voice nattering away in my mind was difficult, so I went to a psychiatrist. As soon as I told him about Dad's illness and the six-year intervals between breakdowns, he diagnosed me as Manic-Depressive. It had taken twenty-four years. He gave me lithium, the treatment approved for MDP at the time, and I threw up twelve times that evening. That was the one and only day in my life I ever took medication for my mental illness.

I shouldn't disparage medication. It has been a boon to many who have led quite normal lives because of it. But I just thank my stars I was ill before they had it. In its stead, I had good old-fashioned psychiatrists. Nothing could take their place.

So what is this book about? About a girl with MDP and too many personalities fumbling her way through life until she was able to contribute a few years to service in the psychiatric field? Perhaps it is, but I prefer to think the book is about that enlightened time when our province was willing to spend so much to help the mentally ill. I remember the day my friend Gwyn exulted, "We're here! At the centre of the universe. We're where it's all happening!" Our hospital didn't win that achievement award just because of the research that was going on. We won because the hospital had moved so rapidly from being a benighted custodial care institution into a modern, humane, progressive hospital offering every kind of therapy. And it was free. Saskatchewan was a model then.

If only we could recapture that spirit: those days of asking and probing and experimenting and trying and helping and caring were taking us to a place where so much satisfaction, so much hope, could be found. The fifties and early sixties were a glory day for psychiatry and for psychiatric patients, and for those who worked in the field. I feel so lucky to have been part of it for a little while.

TOPPLING A MONUMENT

Our mental hospital—the Saskatchewan Hospital at Weyburn—was the pride of its founders, the people of our province. Local citizens loved to motor through the spacious grounds on a Sunday afternoon and brag to visitors about the broad, cool lawns, the happy flowerbeds, the acres and acres of hedge and tree, all cultivated and raked meticulously clean. Gangs of patient workers had planted and maintained those grounds, and patients had literally furnished the hospital. The mattresses on which they slept were made by patients. Hundreds of wicker chairs which lined the wards were made by patients. Patients had prepared rinks, ball diamonds, and tennis courts. The very paintings that hung on the walls had been done by a patient. Patients worked on the hospital farm, which supplied much of their food, and patients did the laundry, scrubbed the corridors, and carried out the garbage. In short, it was a Protestant-ethic hospital.

The main building, vintage early 1920s, was fortunate in its architecture. Its long, low lines were in exquisite proportions and it was graced by a pillared portico over the entrance. Above all that, it was domed, a touch which gave it some of the distinction of the houses of parliament. It was not large, as mental hospitals go, and when the population peaked in the 1930s the count was only 2500. It was gradually reduced until in the late 1950s it was 1500, but since the building had been planned to house 800 patients it was not under-crowded. The wards were large, housing up to 120 people, who slept bed-to-bed in dismal high-ceilinged dormitories that prevented suffocation but permitted a disastrous noise level. The enormous dining rooms clattered their way through an endless series of meals, which had to be eaten in shifts.

The hospital was said to have been a quiet, decent place in the 1920s, before the crowding, but it had had a bad reputation for two decades. In the pre-tranquilizer days there had been much violence, and much coercion. Hundreds of patients were on wards where the only furnishings were heavy wooden benches. They saw no colour, no pictures, no mirrors or curtains or flowers. They had no access to their own clothing or personal possessions. If they were considered dangerous, staff treated them with a mixture of militarism and fear, often with brutality. It was a human garbage heap, and professionals did their best to skim the most promising patients off the top of the heap, give them treatment, and get them out of the place before they, too, began to rot. The burden on the conscience was heavy and staff morale depended not on constructive effort and pride in accomplishment but upon erratic bursts of fun. Staff broke rules, enjoyed a fair amount of immoral conduct, clowned on stage in concerts for the patients, made fun of any patient who might provoke a laugh, and tried to raise their spirits in other non-professional ways. The administration tried to curb these abuses, as insubordination is always curbed— with more rules to be broken.

Yet within that authoritarian milieu, in the midst of odours, ignorance, danger, and din, good people were working, learning to understand mental illness, to tolerate it, and to try to help. The training program for staff kept growing longer, until in the late forties it became a three-year course in psychiatric nursing, and psychiatric nursing became a separate and registered profession in Saskatchewan. The trainees gradually discovered hope and motivation, and a whole range of ideas about relating to the mentally ill. They removed psychiatric nursing from the stigma of "custodial care" or the role of prison guard and pushed it to a new level. They believed that psychiatric nursing was a distinct profession and that no other could claim exact par with it; they discovered professional pride.

Then Dr. Humphry Osmond—the man who gave LSD to Aldous Huxley, which led to Huxley writing *The Doors of Perception* and *Heaven and Hell*—took over the superintendency of the hospital. He walked on to the wards to make his first official rounds and the staff stood to attention, as they always did, and then hastened to unlock the doors for him.

"Please don't get up for me if you're talking to a patient," he said. "Your patient is the important person in this hospital. I can unlock my own doors."

Practically overnight, the ideals the staff had learned in lectures became possibilities. The hospital set about bringing itself out of the middle ages and into the twentieth century. During the fifties, we watched remodelling, replacement of obsolete equipment, and a general facelifting, coupled with an awakening of attitudes and a strong emphasis on research. Dr. Osmond was not only humanitarian, he was creative, and the year (1957) finally arrived when our hospital was named the most improved mental hospital in North America. It might not have been the best, but it was improving by leaps and bounds.

The general public found it hard to adjust to our new administration, because housekeeping began to slip and the grounds, once a tourist attraction, were a mess. Although work is excellent therapy for the mentally ill, the new superintendent believed that if a patient is put to labour *for no pay* it is defined as slave labour, which it is, and he could find no way to rationalize it, which is impossible, and so the grounds were allowed, deliberately, to lapse into disarray. It was amusing, in a bitter way, how interested the public could be in the mental hospital. Many knew that, despite the improvements, there were still far pleasanter places to be, and they shuddered at the thought of ever having to spend a night in it—but they were reluctant to see it changed. They wanted to keep that gold brick facade, surrounded by its lovely grounds, as a monument. They never stopped to think that in erecting their monument they had buried 1,500 people inside it.

The original plan was flouted, at last, by the removal of the dome. It was determined that the old attic was a total waste of space, unheated, and useful only for storage and bats, so it came off to make way for a whole new modern floor. Try as they might, nobody could get very nostalgic about a monument with no dome. I found, personally, that I could live without the dome. What hurt me was that the hedges and flowerbeds, which had made a charming garden at the front door, were demolished in favour of a parking lot. Not even a mental hospital was to furnish a retreat from the encroachment of the modern world, it seemed.

THE NAMELESS THREATS

For many years I had thought vaguely that something was wrong with me, and while studying first-year psychology at college I began to find symptoms of serious mental disorder. Friends just laughed at the idea, but I was beginning to see that the inner life of others didn't contain so much frustration and disillusionment. My father had been in a mental hospital since I was six years old. I had seen him briefly once, when I was seven, and I lived in secret dread that his mental illness might be hereditary. My mother wouldn't talk about him because she believed children should be allowed to forget. I was an only child, with no one else to talk to.

After a year at college I returned to teaching school for a year, and then attended Lorne Greene's Academy of Radio Arts in Toronto in answer to a life-long urge to learn about acting. I had graduated and was working as a secretary at CBC when my life unravelled. Life on a shoestring in a competitive atmosphere led to a crisis. At first it was as if parts of my brain that had been dormant suddenly "awoke" and I became interested in a wide assortment of people, events, places, and ideas that normally would have made no impression on me. Not knowing that I was ill, I made no attempt to understand what was happening, but felt that there was some overwhelming significance in all this, produced either by God or Satan. The walk of a stranger on the street could be a 'sign' to me, which I must interpret. Every face in the windows of a passing streetcar would be engraved on my mind, all of them concentrating on me and trying to pass me some sort of message. New significance in people and places was not particularly unpleasant, though it got badly in the way of my work, but the increased significance of the real or imagined *feelings* of people was very painful. To feel that the stranger passing on the street knows your innermost soul is disconcerting. My mind convinced me that other people had intense feelings towards me—feelings of love, hate, indifference, spite, friendship. These certainties were groundless and led me into dreadful relationships with people. Voices told me I shouldn't eat or sleep, and "forced" me to walk miles and miles about the city until my feet were blistered and bleeding. I was persuaded to do an increasing number of senseless things, but there was no letup in the vicious thoughts that tortured my imagination. Visual and tactile hallucinations began to enliven the auditory ones.

Work in a situation like that is too difficult to be endured. I withdrew farther from reality, but I became more and more aware of the city around me. The real or imagined poverty and real or imagined unhappiness of hundreds of people I would never meet burdened my soul, and I felt martyred. I reached a stage where almost my entire world consisted of tortured contemplation of things that brought pain and unutterable depression. My brain became sore with a real physical soreness. Meaningful distractions from the real world, such as the need to carry on a conversation with a friend, sometimes brought welcome relief from the pain and depression, but not always. I reached a stage of "wakefulness" when the brilliance of light on a windowsill or the colour of blue in the sky would be so important it could make me cry. I had very little ability to sort the relevant from the irrelevant. The filter had broken down. Completely unrelated events became intricately connected in my mind.

I spent two unhappy months and a couple of weeks of living hell in Toronto before my mother realized that something was wrong and flew down to take me home and put me in hospital. Though I fought the idea of hospital restrictions desperately, I experienced a sense of relief as well, knowing that I might be afforded some protection from the nameless threats outside in the world.

PSYCHIATRIC PATIENT

In the summer of 1948 I had a complete mental collapse and ended up at Weyburn. (In later years, I would joke that they'd have to tear the place down if it wasn't for my family.) At the time, I thought it was the tragedy of my life. Actually, I thought it was the end of my life, but it turned out to be the best thing that ever happened. It made me grow up. It gave me insight. It led me into a worthwhile career. Best of all, it opened the door on two of the great mysteries which had haunted me all those years. At last I would find out if my father and grandfather were still thinking human beings. The oppressive fear that had blighted my entire life was about to be lifted.

☙❧

My attention is focused on the morning sunlight coming through the big windows in the day room. It picks out the warmest tones in the red checkers the skinny woman with grey hair is moving about. My senses are enhanced since my breakdown; things look sharper and brighter. Smells are stronger, sounds invasive. My head has been sore for months; so sore it feels as if it has been scoured with sandpaper on the inside. It is very bad today, as I force it to cope with the new setting, the new people, the disillusionment and despair of finding myself in The Big Mental, and with a whole network of shattered dreams. The hopeless weight of the depression is so heavy I can't distinguish the "sensible" voices in my mind from the ones that torment and confuse me.

Despite confusion, I can read the reality of my situation clearly. Perhaps I should say I can grasp it intuitively but I have difficulty putting it into words. A month of treatment at the psychiatric ward in the general hospital, including some electro-shock, has left me jangled, but I know I have only to lose control of my nerves and I could be the one getting the needle. Displease the wrong nurse at the wrong time and I could find myself blacklisted as "troublesome." I have seen patients dragged off to seclusion or, worse, to the notorious basement. I share the fear and frustration known to all of the world's people who live without freedom.

My clothing has come back from being marked with my name, so, respectably clothed, I am sent to eat breakfast in the dining room. A girl named Lillian has befriended me and there is nothing wrong with her but alcoholism, so I have a well-orientated companion to pilot me through the system. Alone, I think I'd die.

We have no trays and the patients who are serving slop porridge all over the sides of our bowls. A piece of toast and a cut orange are plunked on top of the porridge and a plastic cup of milky coffee shoved into my right hand. We sit down at the nearest table across from a row of patients who eat with their hands, mixing orange and toast into the porridge and slurping like dogs. I can't bear the thought of eating.

"Cheer up," says Lillian, "The first seven years are the worst."

At this moment, she couldn't have said a more unfortunate thing if she'd tried. I attempt a smile, but it is sickly. I become aware of a presence beside my chair and for a startled instant I expect a patient to snatch my food.

Then a kindly voice asks, "Would you and Lillian like to come and eat at our table?" It is Mrs. Thomson. I met her yesterday, when I had my hair done at the patient's beauty parlour. She did the shampoo.

We accept her invitation gratefully and are soon seated at a clean table tucked between a window and the servers. There are four middle-aged ladies there, all parole patients with privileges that extend not only to the grounds but even as far as downtown. Each carries a shopping bag bursting with valuables: bread tins, butter jars, sugar jars, and jam jars, to be replenished from the dining-room supplies whenever they run low. They offer to go shopping for us, but make it clear it is illegal to carry mail. They would lose parole if caught posting letters for other patients.

In the dizzying whirl of our rescue, as I learn all this encouraging information, Mrs. Thomson tells me they are friends of my Dad.

All four smile when she says that, even the one who looks ill-tempered. Yes, they've known Dad for many years. He digs their gardens for them in the spring and often helps to weed and water. He built a locked cupboard to hold their tools and canning supplies. These parole ladies even can vegetables. I'm glad to hear they repay Dad for helping them by giving him produce. Dad always loved raw peas and carrots, onions, and tomatoes. I don't have many clear memories of the long-ago time when Dad was at home, but I remember that. He even liked raw potatoes and raw turnips. I'm happy to hear he's had those treats through the long years in hospital.

Obviously, some of the old-timers know how to carve out a home-away-from-home in the place.

"There are some creepy men around these grounds," they tell me, "So we feel safer when your Dad's around. He's cleaned up on some of the bad fellows in his day, and they're afraid of him. But he would never hurt anybody decent. He's a real gentleman, your Dad."

So I haven't been invited to this haven in the corner of the dining room simply on my own merit: my father has paved my way. For eighteen years I've not seen my Dad, and my mother never talked about him. If I ever thought of him, I worried about the condition of his mind, and that produced so much dread I usually tried not to think of him at all. And now he is being presented to me as a reasoning, useful, kindly good neighbour and a "real gentleman."

SUNDAY

Real as the situation is, I have to work to keep focused. Listening to endless inner voices has left my head sore as a lacerated wound. A kind of black curtain separates me from the future, making it impossible to plan. The shock of being in The Mental is the final blow. They brought my father here when I was a child and I never saw him again. My entire life has been shadowed by this hospital, this illness.

It is Sunday. Patients who spend weekdays working in the laundry or sewing room are on the ward, so it is crowded and noisy. The lady who looks like a cross between a ghost and a kindergarten teacher is going out for the day with her family. I wonder if I will ever be allowed a privilege like that, but it is too much to hope for. I return to darkness.

Unless you have experienced deep psychotic depression, I doubt if I can find the words to let you understand the blackest time. It is like being in a tunnel inside a mountain, crawling until exhaustion only to come to a solid wall. "Hopeless" does not cover the situation. Neither does "despair."

I need two things, but I hardly dare admit them to myself. I need to believe my doctor when he says I can recover and leave hospital, and I need to believe the sticky shadows will dissolve and I will actually experience joy again. The worst time of my life was the month I spent in Munro Wing, the psychiatric ward of the General Hospital in Regina. Of course I shouldn't blame the environment entirely, because my frame of mind was down in the pits at that time, but being closed up in a small unit in a city made me feel as if I was in prison. When they told me I was to be transferred down here, I expected much worse—dungeons and cells at least. Instead, I was led through the impressive front door into a wide corridor where the "golden stair" with the wrought-iron railing soared aloft. I found high ceilings, enormous windows. I couldn't go out at first, but I could at least stand at those windows and see the countryside. The Saskatchewan prairie is like the sky, it just keeps on expanding clean up to God. I thought, "People should be able to get well here."

A nurse steps up and asks me to come to church. Church? The sudden hope that I might be taken down town fades promptly. Church will be here in hospital, in the assembly hall. Salvation Army today. As a member of a mainline denomination, I have never been to any church but my own. All I know of the Salvation Army is that they help the poor and sing on street corners to collect funds and save souls.

I demur, but the nurse refuses to take a "No." It would be "good for me" to go to church, so to church I will have to go. About a dozen women are visiting the washroom and tidying their hair, preparing to leave. Catholics don't have to come. We wait for the nurse to unlock doors and we file through the long corridors. Eventually we are all seated left of the aisle, the "female side," toward the back of the assembly hall. Two nurses stand guard at the door to make certain we stay put. The hall stinks of poor personal hygiene. The woman beside me keeps giving deep sighs. A man right of the aisle makes periodic cries that might be "hallelujah's."

On stage, people move at random. I am used to some predictable ritual in a service. I try to feel as if I am in a real church but I can't. I watch the uniformed people shifting places so freely, and I study their individual faces. At least the breakdown has left me the ability to really see. There is a prayer, but mostly they sing, and I don't know any of their songs so I feel alien. That's not unusual; I feel alien to everything in the world. I wonder what kind of faith could help me find hope in this utter gloom.

With their characteristic lively beat, the little band of Army members strike up, *There are shadows in the valley, but there is sunshine on the hill!* I have never heard the song, that I can recall, but my chained spirit reacts by breaking free without warning and starting to soar. The song has cut through my depression so keenly I actually feel my heart opening. There's a tingling I remember as a normal sensation in my brain. My inner voice is exulting, "You will get up there. You will reach the sunshine on the hill."

That moment took a life that had been thrown on the human garbage heap and started it on the long steep climb to the sunshine.

CHRISTMAS COMES TO THE MENTAL

L illian and I are sitting on our narrow cots in the crowded dormitory, debating whether Christmas will come to the mental hospital. It's nearly December and I'm convinced the closest we'll get to Christmas is if they play carols on the radio and the nurses forget to turn it off. Lillian is trying to persuade me Christmas will come, even here. She reminds me the hospital has a fund they use to buy a gift for every patient in the building—all 2000 of them—but I can't believe her. Maybe I don't feel as hopeless or as confused as I did four months ago when I was first admitted, but I'm a long way from happy. The doctor tells me the voices I hear are coming from my own mind and I don't have to listen to them, but it doesn't make any logical sense to me that my own mind would tell me it's God, and single me out for martyrdom, and prophesy all the dreadful things that are supposed to happen to me.

Lillian is in a buoyant mood, so she attempts to brighten my despair by descending upon a potted aster and announcing we will make it into a Christmas tree. She removes the linings from three packages of her cigarettes and we make silver icicles, lanterns, and stars. Some of our fellow patients catch the mood and soon the spindly aster is decked with everything from earrings to embroidery cotton. Our nurses think it's fun, but when the night supervisor comes around she orders the aster dismantled. When we wake in the morning we find, not Christmas, but the usual grey washroom with its elbow-to-elbow sinks. A few weeks later a prosperous tree is carried into the dayroom and correctly decorated with store-bought tinsel and plastic balls. Unlike the aster, it conforms.

My time is being spent in the occupational therapy room these days. I'm told I can feel lucky they didn't put me to work in the laundry. Most of the patients who come to occupational therapy (OT) are old-timers who sit screaming at hallucinatory enemies. They're not very good-natured. Fortunately, the occupational therapist has decided my shock-shattered brain isn't doing such a wonderful job of embroidery that I can't be spared to paint a picture for her, so I've been given the luxury of a worktable of my own. Now they want more paintings for sale at the patients' bazaar, so I'm doing watercolours based on photos in a Scottish calendar. It's something like being in a church group. I do the work and any money it makes goes to the fund. I'm well enough to be clear about the difference between paid employment and slavery. Though I can rationalize selling the embroidery, it rankles to have to give away a God-given talent like my art.

Still, it feels good to paint again. Right after the shock treatments, I couldn't even draw straight. It's hard to select a worst day of my life, but I think the day at Munro Wing when I found I couldn't draw has a very good chance of winning. I had been given electroconvulsive therapy and was outside with a small group of patients and two nurses. One of the nurses handed me a pad of paper and a pencil and asked me to draw—and I couldn't. I had studied art for four years and my first job had been as a commercial artist, but I could not draw. The shocks must have blocked the impulses between the right and left hemispheres. I only know I was aware that I couldn't draw and I believed my skill was gone forever. All those years of work, all the hopes and triumphs had been stolen from me. It would be hard for me to isolate a day more filled with bitterness and despair than that. And I couldn't even talk about it—my skill with words was damaged too. But it has come back in the OT room, where I'm painting watercolours for the bazaar, and I know the relaxation and sense of accomplishment that comes from concentrating on a painting. I'm a firm believer in art therapy.

I try to think altruistic thoughts and concentrate hard enough to shut out the persistent inner voices as they wage war for airtime against the cries of the ladies who sit at their table stitching and cursing. Every so often the therapist says "Sssh," to one of them, reminding her she's too loud. The therapist is kind, strict, and unimaginative.

The OT room is small, tucked into a corner of the fourth-floor attic of the hospital, and sometimes I wonder if anyone in the world knows where we are.

Neil McCallum walks in. Neil's a second-year student of psychiatric nursing. He's a nice-looking boy, though not handsome, with a large, mobile mouth, bright eyes, curly hair, and a nose to rival Cyrano. He's on duty, wearing his white coat over black pants and carrying his keys. Neil never has his keys on his key chain, which is probably why he's always losing them and being reprimanded for it. The therapist asks if he's looking for something.

"I came to get Kay Parley," he says. "We're starting work on the Christmas concert and I need her."

"You can't have her!" she snaps.

For a moment my heart sinks and then I realize she's trying to be funny.

The recreational staff know I'm a graduate of Lorne Greene's Academy of Radio Arts. They've convinced my doctor the best therapy for me would be acting as assistant director for the Christmas entertainment. Neil has permission to spring me from OT.

What a climax to my ambitions—helping stage a concert in a mental hospital. I was working at CBC when it all began, when I stopped going to work because I had to stay home and listen to the voices. Toronto to Weyburn was a bad enough jolt, and now I'm faced with reality: I'm not going to be a professional actress. I'm going to help stage a patients' concert.

Still, the fact there's to be a concert changes my outlook a little. I've been so sure the joyous season would never penetrate these dismal corridors. I go meekly out with Neil but I'm not sure I can be of any use to him. I've lost my confidence and my flexibility. I'm distracted, harried by voices, exhausted and emaciated. I'm in a space without future or purpose. The worst thing about being depressed is this loss of future. I feel I'm doomed to spend eternity locked up in the OT room, and the sudden change they've just made in my routine raises my emotional barometer a few degrees. Neil raises it still more, because he's a warm, stimulating person who insists everything be fun, but at the same time he has sensitivity, and that makes me feel understood.

When we reach the assembly hall I meet Irene Russon. She's wearing her uniform, keeping an eye on a small band of patients who are her responsibility because they don't have parole. I don't have parole either, because I've threatened to run away or commit suicide. It doesn't seem to worry Neil or Irene. They are the kind of people who go by intuition.

Tiny, blonde, and sharp-featured, Irene reminds me of Marlene Dietrich. She has the least respect for bureaucratic systems of anyone I ever met and that's good for me, too, because I've just spent sixteen weeks being ground down by one of the most repressive bureaucracies ever known.

Irene's complaining that the nurse who promised to bring the music has forgotten and I tell her I have some in my locker. Irene's thinking fast. She looks over the group of non-parolees and she knows she can't leave the hall. Neil has gone to collect a few men from one of the wards so, from the staff's point of view, Irene is "alone." Suddenly she whisks her keys off her belt, turns, and hands them to me.

"Go let yourself on the ward and get the music," she says, "And if you meet anybody, swallow the keys."

A nurse can be fired on the spot for handing her keys to a patient. Irene's trust, not to mention her daring, gives me a sense of responsibility I haven't felt in months. My feet feel light for the first time since my admission.

It looks as if I may be in for the first tolerable time I've found in the hospital. Mind you, we're not very professional. The most talented member of our troupe can do a step dance and another plays a squeaky fiddle, but if it doesn't bother Neil and Irene it doesn't bother me. We're actually having fun. I'm in on all the decision-making and I'm working with two people who insist I be a person, not a patient. The ward nurses always make it clear they have superior status around here and patients are only patients. The recreational staff set such distinctions aside. For the first time, I'm able to relax.

My new role brings new contacts, and soon I'm helping to design the next issue of the hospital newspaper, *The Torch*. They ask me to do a drawing for the cover that can be cut into a stencil. It gives me an idea.

Somewhere in the hospital, my father is living. I haven't seen Dad since they brought him here eighteen years ago. Twice I've asked my doctors if I can see him and the answer is, "Not yet." I can't understand their reluctance. I have friends among the old ladies who are trustees, and they know my Dad. They've assured me he's well respected and they can't see "anything wrong with him," but they all believe they're sane, so I don't know what to think.

I want to send some kind of tangible message to Dad, and here's my chance. I draw my grandfather's stone house, the home where my Dad grew up. Pictured among snow banks, the two fir trees burdened with winter, it's the ideal cover for the Christmas *Torch*. Now all I can do is wait. I'm learning what the old-timers mean by being "smart." I don't even tell Neil and Irene what the sketch depicts, but let Dad get a look at the next paper and he'll know I'm in my right mind.

Our rehearsals are usually in the afternoon, but as Christmas draws nearer we're often in the hall after supper, working as late at 8:30. That's past bedtime on most wards. One night, after the others have gone, Neil asks Irene and me back to his ward for coffee. Irene wants to know who my charge-nurse is on that shift and, when she hears it's a friend of hers, she says, "Easy!" She phones the ward to say, "Kay will be late. We need her for a conference. I'll have her back by ten."

These two rule-breakers have just boosted me up another big step. It bothers me a little, being overly conscientious since my breakdown, that it's taking a bit of larceny to free me from the bonds of mental illness, but it's obviously working. How long has it been since I sat up until ten o'clock chatting over coffee? We talk about Saskatchewan winters and country schools, the dirty thirties and my radio ambitions. I feel nervous about telling them I'd dearly love to meet my father, and when I bring the subject up they're the ones who look nervous.

"I have to know how he is," I explain. "Worrying about that has been a strain for me all my life. All the doctor tells me is I don't have what he has."

Neil quickly agrees with the doctor. Neil and Irene are exchanging glances and finally Irene admits that the doctors are adamant about my not meeting my father until I am well. They think it will be emotionally tough on me.

So my new friends don't think I'm well.

I have to fight to hold back tears. What is wrong with these people? Don't they know it's emotionally tough on me just wondering? Not knowing? I simply can't understand. Still, there's something constructive about the incident. I feel almost normal at the coffee party. I know my doctor is always behind the scenes, supervising every step of my treatment, but Neil and Irene seldom remind me of that. I'm part of the team, working on the show.

It seems there's never a happy time in the hospital that isn't interrupted by a setback. The next morning I've got severe pain in my ribs, and the doctor thinks it's pleurisy and puts me on sick ward. Great! Here I am without stimulation, save for the whimpering of the senile and the sickening redolence of bedsores. I figure I'll miss the concert and end up back on OT listening to the ladies curse. When I pray, my inner voice reminds me, *God helps those who help themselves.*

"How can I help myself when I have no control over anything that happens to me?" I fume.

You have control over your thoughts, says the voice. *You have control over your state of mind.*

The doctor decides I don't have pleurisy. What I have is shingles, and all I need is a rest. I'm sent back to the admitting ward and allowed to languish in bed in the empty dorm, surrounded by twenty-three little white cots, with the bleak winter light silvering the ceiling-high windows that line one side of the room. The windows are deceptively barred. The frames around the small panes look like wood but they're bars, or so I've been told.

When I first came to the hospital I stood at one of those windows and gazed out on a bright autumn day. I noted how lovely nature looked and how close-minded and miserable some of the nurses looked and how out-of-it some of the patients looked, and I asked myself, *Which side of the fence is the prison on?* It struck me you could only be in prison if you put yourself in one. If I left my mind out there in the sunshine, I could be out there too. I didn't have to be in here. Not my soul.

As I'm thinking these thoughts, Neil McCallum walks in. He's carrying two large wire frames, scissors, thread, cheesecloth, and yards of tinsel.

"Get to work," he says, "and trim your wings for the concert."

I've agreed, after quite a bit of persuasion, to appear in the concert as the Christmas angel.

Now, I'm thinking triumphantly, as I busy myself with swathy cheesecloth and bright tinsel, *Which side of the fence is the prison on?* When I'm relaxed, the supportive voice is with me, the one I call my "true love." I'm in harmony today. Rehearsals are still being held but I had the show memorized long ago, so I'm not afraid of missing anything.

All the activity has prompted me to ask my doctor for parole and I've got it—not free parole or even grounds parole, but parole within the building, which is the next best thing. No more waiting for a nursing escort. On the day of the concert I'm able to walk without pain, if I'm careful, and I can walk free. I have my hair done at the patients' beauty parlour and head for the hall.

In the main corridor, I meet the patient nobody trusts. I've been warned to stay away from him because he's never honest and he lives, it seems, to try to get female patients pregnant. He always asks me to dance, and he appears to treat me with respect. I've heard that my father has a reputation for being able to defend himself. Maybe it's occurred to some of these guys that he could also defend his daughter.

"I've got a message for you," he says, looking around to be sure no one is within hearing. "Tonight your Dad will be at the concert. I'll sit with him and we'll be on the aisle, about halfway down. Come in that way and I'll introduce you."

Dad must have seen the picture of the stone house! I'm nervous and a little guilty about plotting behind the backs of the authorities, but there's no time to think about that. Neil has lined up a small knot of nurses to go carolling on wards where they have old folks who can't get out to the concert. Neil is dressed as Santa. One of the male nurses plays a mean guitar. My depression begins to recede with the realization there are others worse off than I am. Some patients are able sit up to listen to our music, and a few thank us for coming.

Then we go out into the cold and cross to the TB Annex to take our carols to another group. In the basement of that building is the children's ward. There, in cribs and on low, small cots, are Down's Syndrome children, others with hydrocephalus, all tiny, some dwarfed. They are not all young in years. I feel profound shock as we walk into that ward. I'd been raised in a sheltered home. Before I came to hospital, I knew very little about the people who face these kinds of problems.

The "children" take one look at Santa Claus and react like children anywhere. There are hysterical squeals and excited laughter. Some are bounding on their beds so high they fall. Others run to hug Santa, and a few of them hug us all. They love the music and we sing more for them than we did for the others, they're so appreciative.

My wings are on stage waiting for me, but I get into my costume on the ward and cover it with my coat when it's time to go down for the concert. My young acquaintance is seated on the aisle as he promised, and beside him is a handsome man with wavy grey hair and a jaunty set to his broad shoulders that I'd almost forgotten. He's older, yes, but it's my Dad. I'm not sure what I expected. A thin, tragic, white-skinned, babbling wreck, I guess. I've seen hundreds like that in the hospital. I don't know very much about manic-depressive psychosis.

Dad stands up with all the dignity he can command and looks at me with those clear blue eyes I remember and holds out his hand. A Scotsman doesn't hug or kiss, especially not in a hall already three-quarters full of people. He shakes my hand and I have a Dad again, after eighteen years. I'd forgotten the vitality in his voice.

It's true! He isn't a wreck at all. I'm so excited I'm flying. When I get to the stage I blurt it out to Neil: "I just met my father!"

Neil looks scared, but it isn't his fault. He says, "I hope this isn't going to set you back. You've been doing so well."

"How could meeting my father possibly set me back?"

I don't know much about the impact of old ties, old emotions. I think the excitement is anticipation, but perhaps there is some anxiety. In any event, it turns out okay. I cope with meeting my father very well.

Neil has done his best to make it a good show. Once I'm into my wings and the chorus is formed, he leads us out the stage door, down a ramp to the hospital basement, up a flight of steps and through the entry hall to the back of the auditorium. We will enter from the rear, singing as we come, and we expect it to make an impression. I will lead down centre aisle (where Dad and I can exchange another grin) and at the front I will turn right and lead them down the side of the hall, across the back and up the left aisle to the stage. If "O Come All Ye Faithful" isn't long enough to take us all the way, we'll begin "Hark The Herald Angels Sing."

I adjust my halo. Irene begins to play.

The women patients always sit on one side of the centre aisle, the men on the other, and the men are usually quieter, the ones most down-beaten, the ones most drawn into themselves. As I lead the chorus around the male side of the hall, the sad faces look up at me, grey and lined with the emotional disturbance of years, eyes confused or dead or bright with wild delusions. An angel should love, and so I try to project some kind of heavenly love, but it's difficult. The thick air assaults me, the usual heavy mix of urine and sweaty feet, strong laundry soap and old clothes. The shock of the mental hospital has hit me hard.

I still feel that sense of revulsion, hoping I won't accidentally brush close to any of the patients as I go by. I can't imagine how the nurses manage to touch these people.

Irene is trying to pick up the beat, see if the singers can be persuaded to go a little faster. Certainly one or two of our angels are slow and some are out of tune or sliding off the notes, and yet these voices, plucked from wards all over the hospital, sound rich and joyful tonight. The sound goes up to the high ceiling and reflects back as a thing of beauty.

I swing right and, at the second turn, a long-term patient is seated, muttering to himself. He is a broken specimen of mankind, untidy, the kind I find repulsive. I doubt if he knows where he is, but he reaches out his hand and touches my robe, gently, as if he expects it to melt away. There's an expression of awe on his face, like a child who has found something marvellous under the tree. He has really seen a Christmas angel.

MEETING GRANDPA

When I was born I had a Grandma Dyer living at Fleming, but no Grandpa Dyer. I remember being puzzled about that. Mother told me Grandpa was in a hospital. No, he wasn't going to die, but he wasn't coming home. It was a poser for a child. As the years went by, I learned my grandfather was in the mental hospital, and I wasn't to ask questions until I was older.

When that day came, Mother explained that Grandpa had "lost control of his nerves" and reached the stage where he couldn't preach. The family were living at McLeod, Alberta, when Grandpa had to give up the pulpit. Of all the towns where they had lived (a Methodist minister automatically moved every three years), Grandma liked Fleming best, so Grandpa bought her the big square house on the hill at Fleming, and that became the Dyer home. In 1921, soon after the mental hospital at Weyburn opened, J.D. Dyer was admitted as a patient. The hospital, big, clean and airy, was considered one of the best of its time and was purported to be a fairly nice place in the twenties. The two wings that existed at the time had an 800-patient capacity and it was not over-crowded.

Mother made no secret of the fact she was bitter about her father. She hated anything that disturbed her routine and he had been a disturbing factor. She criticized him for "losing his head in an emergency" and she resented him because Grandma had to work so hard and bear so many children. She thought him chauvinistic, "though not as bad as some men of that day and age." It was many years before my mother told me what had turned her so against her father, and it was easy to understand.

It had to do with her little sister Vera, who had died just as she turned three. Vera was a highly intelligent child who sparkled with love and the joy of living. Grandfather doted on her, and he was not alone in that. Mother adored that baby sister. She thought she was the luckiest girl in the world to look forward to a lifetime with a sister like that. Then Vera died of spinal meningitis. Grandma, believing it best not to talk things over with children (because it was kinder to let them forget), gave Mother no sympathy. Grandpa did far worse. In the midst of his grief, he gestured to Mother and said, "Why couldn't it have been this one?"

So Mother had to cope with her dreadful loss without support, and take this brutal rejection on her father's part on top of it—and she was only seven. It is easy to see why she found it almost impossible to forgive.

In spite of the bitterness, Mother was always quick to give her father credit for his good points. She admitted that he was still a "human being" when she and her oldest brother were very small. She said, "He was interested in us. He seemed to enjoy getting to know us and teaching us things. He was highly intelligent and well read, and it was a treat to have a real talk with him. He had tremendously high ideals and never made any secret of the fact that he expected a lot of us, but that never bothered us. We were ambitious too."

Mother also talked a lot about her father's charitable ideals, though she did feel it was unfair that he used their house as a kind of welfare centre without seeming to realize it all meant more work for his wife. Mother had a strong identification with her mother, possibly because, as the oldest daughter, she got a huge share of the work and childcare. Despite the deaths of Vera and the little brother who came next in line, there were still six younger siblings in the family.

What troubled Mother most was her father's complete dominance in the home: "I seldom saw Mother get her way. She was too busy trying to keep our father's temper in line. She didn't want to antagonize him, but how she kept so pleasant and good-humoured herself I really don't know."

If I grew up with an image of this grandfather I had never seen, it was probably one of style. He had a deep appreciation of quality and he liked it to show. He loved to be decked out in a good buggy with a fast driving team, and he cut a fine figure driving them. He dressed to his own sense of taste and status. Mother said, "I never saw him looking sloppy."

Mother's most positive feelings about her father centered around that sense of good taste. When she left home to attend Normal School, her father took her shopping and bought her the best leather suitcase they could find. It was the sort of bag no one would want nowadays because it weighed about twenty-five pounds empty, but it was glorious cowhide with sturdy straps, and it just glowed. Her father said, "Always buy the best, Merle. There is no substitute for quality. Nothing else is worth the money."

Mother went on to say, "It was the one thing, I think, that I really had in common with my father, that same love of quality."

Growing up like that, occasionally hearing a word or two about my grandfather but never knowing him,

I resisted thinking about him very much. If I did any ruminating about such things, my thoughts were more likely to centre on my Dad.

When I was in Weyburn and asked to meet my Dad, they said "no" at first, believing the meeting should be postponed until I had my head together. I didn't ask to meet my grandfather. Why should I? I'd never known him. I had no reason to believe he'd know who I was. But a mental hospital is like a big village—gossipy. The hospital grapevine buzzed all the time. I heard that my grandfather had a private room on one of the quietest wards in the hospital. I heard he had free parole and could come and go as he pleased, that he often went for a walk in the morning before breakfast. I heard that Grandfather read a lot and that he had always skated. In fact, he had taught many of the patients in the hospital to skate. Best of all, I heard from my doctor that my grandfather was "the most respected patient in this hospital." That was made obvious by the fact nobody called him Jabez or J.D. In a place where even grey-haired grandmothers were often called by their first names, my grandfather was referred to as "Reverend Dyer." He had spent many years working in the tailor shop, where they made clothing for male patients, but he was now retired.

I took in all this information gratefully. Being a resident in the mental hospital soon taught me that the patients they called paranoid were often well dressed. They were likely to be proud people who walked with good carriage. They conversed normally. They were the ones visitors would point to and ask, "Why is he or she here? I don't see anything wrong with them." The more I learned about Grandpa Dyer and his ilk, the less worried I was that he had deteriorated like so many of the 2,000 patients in the place.

Then came the surprise. My doctor asked me if I would like to meet my grandfather. I said, "I don't think so. I don't imagine he'd know me."

"Oh, he knows you," was the answer. "He has asked to meet you."

I was flattered but I was scared. What would he be like? Would it be upsetting?

"Relax," said the doctor. "Your grandfather is a very fine man. Just don't start to talk about religion or politics. He can get pretty excited about those."

I had no idea what to expect. Mother had painted her father as an erratic, incendiary man, brilliant but emotionally out of control. I pictured him as large. I had seen his photos and I knew he had the big forehead he had passed to many of his children, so I rather thought the rest of him would be big too. But he knew me and he had asked to meet me. What would be expected? Would he want me to hug him?

It is fascinating how memory works. My breakdown had vividly pointed up the almost magical way in which it unfolds, often bringing the most relevant thought to mind at the right time. As I was having a bath and preparing to dress up to meet Grandpa, I suddenly remembered something else my mother had said about her dad.

She said, "I must admit I wanted him to appreciate me. I don't remember wanting him to love me. I don't think I would have dared to think of such a thing, because even Mother didn't love me. Neither of them really knew what love was. They had come of a culture where deportment and moral behaviour counted most. Achievement counted an awful lot, but emotion was not something to discuss or develop. What I did like about Dad was his ability to see us as people, whereas Mother saw us as little under-developed human beings and never seemed to wake up to our uniqueness as personalities until we were grown. And yet she was our balance wheel, our peacemaker, our United Nations, and always our source of cheer. Without her, we would all have gone stark raving insane. We all put a deep love of our mother into the deepest core of our beings and we never lost it. She was practically a goddess in our home."

I knew that gentle, popular, laughter-loving grandmother very well, but the memory did nothing to put me at ease about the kind of man I was about to meet. It did settle the question about hugging. It didn't seem likely I would be expected to be demonstrative, and that pleased me. I had learned to relate best across a table.

A nurse escorted me to the visitors' corridor on the male side, and she timed it well. As we entered the corridor, a small, neat gentleman was ushered through the doors at the other end. He had a cane, less a necessity than a prop, and he was immaculate in a grey suit. He carried a smart tweed cap and told me proudly that day that he had made it in the tailor shop. It was a masterpiece.

The visitors' corridors were just that—long, narrow corridors designed to give families access to patients behind lock and key, in those days when mental hospitals were places of strict control. They had large bays where five tall windows admitted the east light, and comfortable armchairs woven of wicker right there in the hospital. It was not unpleasant.

We shook hands and sat down and appraised each other. I decided I liked my grandfather. I could sense immediately that he had a bright, far-ranging mind. Know me? He knew every grandchild and what they were doing, where they were, who they had married, when (if) they had last come to see him. He talked of my oldest uncle's family with love and interest. He knew I had been at the radio school and started right in to talk to me about plays. No one had ever told me that one of Grandpa's chief interests was drama.

It couldn't be a completely easy visit, not across all that time and all that uncertainty. I felt the immense sadness of a life wasted. He was so close to well, so attached to his own, and he had been bound to this place for twenty-seven years. It was a place with so much ugliness in it, so much that was obscene, and Grandpa was devoted to beauty, scholarship, and goodness. It was what had troubled me most since my own admission—the contrast between the sheltered, almost genteel life for which I had been raised, and the chaos into which I had been pitched. Why? What was God trying to prove? Had Grandpa had some positive influence on the place, even in the role of patient?

I had heard he came here willingly, knowing he didn't function well in the outside world, but I was still smarting about my own hospitalization, so it was hard to understand. Still, the meeting left me with more positive feelings about Grandpa than negative ones, and I visited with him in that corridor several times. When Mother and one of her brothers came to see me, they came to see us both, and took Grandpa out to dinner. After I left the hospital I returned to see him at times, but I always went a little reluctantly. Had there been more people to participate and had we not been in hospital surroundings, I might have felt more at ease. Grandpa had wit and great sensitivity. He prodded me to talk about books I had read. I believe he sensed I had not found my walk in life and he asked leading questions about that. Once I asked him if he still skated and he gave a grin that said, "We all get old." Aloud he said, "Not as much as I used to." He was in his eighties, but he was still skating.

I went to say goodbye to Grandpa when I moved away from Weyburn in 1952, and I never saw him again. I was in Toronto in January, 1955, when Jabez Daniel Dyer died, in the hospital where he had lived for thirty-four years. Grandma had him buried at Calgary, where she was living. When I heard of his death, I cried, and thought how fortunate it was that he hadn't died before we met. Then, he would have been a mere shadow passing. Now he was a loss. My grandfather had become a real person to me and I admired him for the way he had endured all those years in the hospital and kept his integrity, his humanity, and the essential quality of worth that was so important to him. The way in which he won the respect of the mental hospital staff alone says a great deal about Rev. J.D. Dyer.

In many ways, Grandpa was a victim of his times. It was a time when a mother could choose a career for her son, regardless of his temperament, a time when the expectations on a minister were overwhelming, and a day when there was a conspiracy of silence about all emotional and personal matters. There was little communication between husband and wife in most homes, and males were expected to live up to ridiculous standards. Given the same ideals and the same level of education, I would hardly expect a father of the early twenty-first century to blurt out the seven hurtful words J.D. turned on my mother when they lost Vera. If he did, I would expect today's father to realize the damage he had caused and do his best to make amends. My grandfather was born in 1866, in extremely Victorian Ontario. I suppose no era can be considered the best era in which to be alive, but perhaps we are slightly more enlightened today. Mother talked so much about Grandma's patience, and how hard she tried to keep Grandpa calm, but I don't think anyone asked whether Grandpa was getting much understanding or support. Everyone was expected to face up to difficulties, especially the head of a family. As I said, J.D. Dyer was a victim of his times.

He was also the product of his times in a more constructive way. He was of an age when every family strove to be respectable at least, and better than that if possible. High achievement was expected of every bright child. Moral character and good manners were required. During the last fifty years there has been a conscious levelling off, everyone striving for the least common denominator. Pride in dress and behaviour disappeared. High status seems to be a mark of shame, no longer the sign of hard work and success. The quality of excellence as a standard of anything has become obscured. Without goals to achieve, children have lost incentive. Without norms to follow, society has become lax and sloppy and has tried to compensate for these losses by exalting money.

When I was growing up, I always knew my mother's family held themselves in high regard. I thought it was because they were a minister's family, raised to believe they must set the standards. I knew, too, they were aware they had brains, personality, and leadership qualities. I knew Grandma's cheerful dignity inspired respect and that it had great influence on the family. It wasn't until I met Grandpa that I got the rest of the equation. His intelligence, his taste, his flair for showmanship—these were the qualities that had given the family that extra edge.

THE TORCH

Treatment was long-term in the forties. When I had been in the Saskatchewan Hospital at Weyburn for five months I was considered well enough to take over editorship of the in-house paper, *The Torch*. The little 8 × 10 mimeographed publication was due to celebrate its first anniversary in February. I was terrified. How could I possibly organize my wandering thoughts enough to edit a paper? Where would I find the confidence? But I had a little experience as assistant editor on two or three school papers, I had taken a class in writing, I was a commercial artist with experience at a printer's, and I was a typist. When the doctor said it would be good for me, I became editor of *The Torch*.

My new job gave me the illusion of freedom. I had parole, and now I had an office of my own. It was partitioned off at the end of a wide corridor not far from the door to my own ward. The entry to the personnel director's office was beside it, and he acted as staff advisor. An entry to the staff dining room was opposite, so interested staff could easily wander in with ideas and encouragement. Best of all, the location was quiet compared to the ward.

A joint patient-and-staff effort, the paper was supported by a band of four staff reporters, a nurse in charge of circulation, and another of advertising. (Downtown businesses were quite willing to spend a quarter for an ad in our paper). Our directors were a staff advisor and a long-term female patient. One of the assistant editors was a patient. Two patients ran the mimeograph machine, the standard method of duplication in the 1940s for those without a printing press. Much of my day was spent arranging pages and typing them on stencils, doing illustrations with a stylus. The paper always had a coloured cover: pink for February, green for March. Page one listed editorial staff and hospital census, and contained any special communications. January had a note from the superintendent, Dr. Coulter. In February, we ran a congratulatory message from Premier T.C. Douglas, commending us on our first anniversary. Page two carried the editorial. I have no memory of writing the editorial that appeared in the

February edition, and I can't recall who did, but it was not my style. It was an ambitious statement:

"Our Torch would like to spread its light in ever-increasing brightness over a dubious province and country, carrying with it a knowledge and understanding of illness of the mind, of the functions of this great structure of ours and the work necessary among the inhabitants of our community, among patients and staff, and among all those communities which must necessarily prepare to receive and assist those who leave here seeking rehabilitation and a chance to live normally in this world of ours. It is to these citizens abroad that we throw our Torch."

That is only about a quarter of the original editorial, which makes no secret of our ambitions. The people who launched the *Torch* were idealists and they had the secret of therapy: patients had to be included in hospital projects. Staff and patients had to work together if they were to achieve success. *The Torch* waved that banner at every opportunity—that it was a joint staff-patient effort.

Our features included a "Personality of the Month" and "Food for Thought." Pages were devoted to recreational activities, occupational therapy, sports, staff news, and ward news contributed by patients. Mention was made of coming events, such as films, concerts, and church services. There were introductions to new staff, mention of staff who left or patients who were discharged.

The paper ran to twenty pages and sold for five cents a copy or fifty cents a year. Any surplus income went to the patients' bazaar fund, to be used for Christmas or birthday gifts for patients who had no family contacts.

It took all my effort to put out the January issue. By May, I was working full time at a typist's job downtown and editing the paper in my spare time. Such an improvement in five months is proof enough that the *Torch* was therapeutic for patients involved. It is interesting that the most valuable job I ever did paid nothing at all— nothing, that is, except my health, my confidence, and my self-respect.

The big mental hospital was not a mere conglomerate of separate individuals suffering from mental illness. It was a community, a village of over 2,000 people, counting staff, bound by familiar scenes and familiar routines, brightened by welcome surprises. No space was wasted space. If there was an inch to spare, a little editor's note would convey an item of news or perhaps an optimistic nudge from a patient--"Any community can only be as pleasant as the people in it. Help to make our ward a cheerful and happy community. Your life is made up of the friends you make"—contributed by a patient on the female admitting ward.

I spent a week at home in Regina in March that year and saw the movie *The Snake Pit*. Not surprisingly, an article by "a patient" appeared in the next *Torch*, entitled "Is This Hospital a Snake Pit?" I don't suppose many were puzzled by the authorship. Perhaps I was a little too kind to our hospital, tending to ignore the fact that we had several wards which were snake pits indeed, but after all, the place was home. It could be fun, too. For instance, I come upon a note about the male attendants' quarters: "This space has to remain blank, owing to the fact that those queried about their activities display all the earmarks of guilt complexes and refuse to talk!"

The editor of *The Weyburn Review* called the *Torch* "One of the most refreshing papers to reach this desk in a long time. Any publication which is a true representation of the highest aspirations of a group of people merits approval." Old clippings I saved show that we also received favorable mention in the *Western Producer* and the *Kamsack Times*. I don't remember how many papers received copies of the *Torch*, but there is every indication we were out to make mental illness as friendly and familiar as we possibly could. We wanted to present a true picture of life in the hospital, and we wanted to help overcome the stigma attached to mental hospitals and mental hospital patients.

Nine years after my stint as editor, the Saskatchewan Hospital at Weyburn was under new administration and, as mentioned earlier, was named the most improved mental hospital on the continent. By that time, I was training as a psychiatric nurse in the hospital. Since I was then seeing it from another perspective, it is hard to know if my observations are completely correct, but I am still bothered by the feeling that the more professional staff attitudes became, the more distance was created between staff and patients. Attitudes were kinder, there was so much understanding, but the camaraderie that existed between sociable patients and enlightened staff in the old hospital didn't seem to be there any more. The secret, of course, was community. The hospital in the forties, with all its faults, had the feeling of a permanent community. It was a bizarre community, a police state, but it had cohesion, and the *Torch* promoted community.

By asking me to play a creative and responsible role in a project that involved supposedly normal individuals working *with* patients, I was given the opportunity to see myself as a contributing member of society once more. I find it discouraging that the medical model has led psychiatry to a position of "You are sick. I can help you," when what is needed is a sense of "You can help me. You can contribute to the community." That was the magic of the old *Torch*.

THE GLASS OF TRUTH

We are expecting a quiet evening. There is nothing going on in the assembly hall, so Lillian and I plan to wash our hair and go to bed early. Sleep is hard to come by in the noisy, crowded dorms of the mental hospital, so it is a precious thing.

Suddenly the supervisor steps up to me and tells me my doctor wants to see me in the hall. Not his office? No, the assembly hall. I am instructed to dress in my best. The staff are secretive about whatever is going on and I am scared. Everything makes my heart leap these days—even opening a door.

I put on the brown suit Mother made when I set off for the Academy of Radio Arts less than two years ago. It is a fashion called "riding habit," with a gentle flare to the hip-length jacket. My mother is a superb seamstress and it's a smart outfit. I comb my hair and put on makeup and feel that, for someone mentally ill, I look rather well. I have neat brown pumps. When a psychiatrist says, "Be dressed up," I know what he means.

My nurse leaves me at the door of the assembly hall. (Not even a parole patient wanders the hospital corridors alone after supper.) When I see the assemblage, I want to run. There are no patients at all; just staff and outsiders. At first glance it is a forbidding crew, but I notice two young male attendants who have been in skits with me. There is the man I type letters for during the day, a student nurse who's on recreation this shift, my own doctor, somebody's wife I should recognize. In a minute I realize they are all familiar faces: a steno from front office who is always friendly, a young man who works downtown in the health centre, one of the social workers. My anxiety becomes something I can cope with.

They tell me they are all people who like drama, so they have come together to do some ad-lib scenes. My first thought is, "They're forming a drama group and I'm to be in on it!" The idea of being the only patient allowed into the holy precincts of a staff group is heady. Still, my intuition is pricking. There must be more to it than that.

A movement in the balcony catches my eye. It is dark up there, but I can make out two or three figures slipping out from behind the projection booth and taking seats. I promptly ask about them, but my doctor brushes them aside as unimportant. "They're not part of the group. Just curious. Don't pay any attention to them. Pretend they're an audience." But you do pay attention to an audience. The little group of curiosity-seekers troubles me.

Chairs have been arranged in a casual circle at the front of the hall, and someone puts on the stage lights. The social worker and the personnel director get up to do the first scene. Setting it up is too simple. It is easy to see they have done some pre-planning before my arrival, and that makes me uncomfortable. It is an unhappy scene about a woman insisting her husband has to go to hospital, while he protests, quite ineffectually, that he is not sick. It reminds me that some such scene must have taken place in my home when Dad was brought here to the hospital. I don't like it.

They ask me to go on stage for the next scene, and I am worried about whether or not I can act. I wish I could see the reactions of those people in the balcony, but they are still in darkness. Our scene is set at a table and I find myself opposite the social worker who is playing my mother. The two of us are alone together—no father, no siblings. Oh oh! I strongly suspect my doctor of playing a game. Well, I can play the game. They tell me to say whatever comes into my head; do whatever occurs to me to do. I do not like the idea of them seeing me in scenes so close to my personal reality, but I will try. I am still struggling to hold to the illusion that they just want to enjoy some play-acting.

The social worker knows that my mother is domineering and that she tends to think she owns me, but her concept is enough out of sync with my mother that I find it disconcerting. She wants to know what I'm doing for the evening. I have been told to tell her I am going on a date, so of course she wants to know where and who with. My mother is the fastest thinker I ever met, and dueling with her is often like dancing. The social worker doesn't dance. I feel as if she's going to drag me into a fight faster than my real mother would. This is the stupidest scene I ever imagined.

Suddenly, she begins to talk about Alex. She is wishing my date was with him. Why did I break up with Alex? How did I really feel about him?

I feel as if I'd been kicked in the stomach. Who told the social worker about Alex? Oh yes, I was complaining to my doctor that my so-called college friends had totally rejected me when I came to the mental hospital. He asked me if there was no one among them who might be concerned enough about me to come and see me, so I said, "Alex might." I must have forgotten that Alex said we could never be friends. So the doctor wrote to Alex and received the letter he handed to me, the letter that wished me well and said it would not be a good idea to come and see me. The letter that said, "I am involved with someone else now." Now I know what they mean when they say tears can sting the eyes, but I am not going to let these people know they have hurt me. I feel betrayed.

"I asked you how you felt about breaking up with Alex."

This is ridiculous. Mother would criticize, she would tell me I should have put more thought into it, but she would never ask me how I felt about it. Emotion is not compatible with Mother's mindset of common sense and duty. Emotions are nothing but trouble and not to be considered. I just don't know how to respond.

"You never ask me something like that."

"Well, I am asking you now. Answer me."

"Answer you? About how I feel? You know how I felt about Alex. He was a nice guy. He was smart. I admired Alex a lot."

"But you threw him over for that useless substitute. He wasn't in it with Alex."

"Mother, I know how you felt about Alex. All I did was flirt with the other guy at the rink and Alex wanted no more to do with me. I thought he was pretty unforgiving."

"That's it? He was 'unforgiving'? You didn't find anything else wrong with him?"

I can't take this any more. I blurt, "His feet were too big. Okay?"

It sounds so shallow. Somewhere in the hall, I hear a titter.

I am saved by the arrival of Neil McCallum, the young attendant I worked with on the Christmas concert. He is playing my date. There is a lot of empathy between us. We are joined at the "restaurant" table by one of the student nurses. Neil introduces me and she says, "Didn't you go with Alex Wray?" Strangely, I feel as if I expected that. I talk about Alex sensibly, but somehow I have walked into a baffling trap. I thought Alex was gone—dropped away into the past—and here he is dominating everything. This "date" is totally spoiled. Then I am back at the home set and "Mother" is asking where we went and reminding me I said I would be home at 10:30 and it is 10:45. I have enough fight left to say, "Mother, I will be twenty-five in two weeks. I know enough to come in at night."

With that, I stalk off "to bed" and I have no intention of letting her drag me into anything more. I stumble from the stage ready to weep, but I am determined not to break down. Neil is waiting for me at the top of the stair, wearing a beaming smile. "You're doing great!" he says, but Neil has a dramatic sensitivity my doctor lacks. He reads my face on the instant and adds, "It isn't fair. They should have warned you."

I nod. Neil's understanding helps me find some kind of balance. I return to my chair feeling like a trembling aspen, but in control.

They bring on the personnel director again, my "father." Is this how they see my father? This dull, unmotivated man without a spark of courage? Is this how Dad shows himself to the staff? It makes me angry. I was only seven when Dad came to hospital, but I do have memories and I know how he was viewed by the folks at home. Dad was an athlete, an extrovert, a man full of laughter and wit who played the fiddle and enjoyed life. He still has a colourful presence, unless he's around the staff who have repressed him all these years. Dad's eyes react to everything, enjoying all the quirks of all the personalities around him. The personnel director is playing him with lifeless eyes. I feel sick.

He asks, "Did you miss me?" and I feel that somewhere deep inside is a bottomless well of tears, but I don't know how to find them. I say, "Miss you? It left me alone with Mother, and she is not always the easiest person in Canada to get along with."

He gives a faint grin. I want to say, "And it meant leaving the farm." Nothing has ever shattered me like leaving the farm, like having no home. But I don't like to say it because, if this was really Dad, it would make him feel bad.

"But did you miss *me*, personally?" he persists. I know Dad wouldn't ask that, but I want to cry. If this was a real actor, I think I would start to sob on his shoulder. My chin is trembling. This man is talking about my Daddy, the person I had cause to miss most in the world. The Daddy I loved best of anyone. But this isn't an actor, it is the personnel director, the man I type letters for these days. And he's staff. I won't play the scene. I can't. I say, "Of course I missed you," and I keep control.

I tell myself it is all coincidence. It isn't my life we are presenting. Maybe they have used my story as a spring-board for the scenes. Maybe they hope to work up a play out of this. Maybe . . . But I know better. I act. I won't let them see my reactions to scenes that touch me so closely.

"Do you think we should take a break?" asks my doctor, and they have cigarettes and chat about how well we are doing. They admit they are getting a bit personal and talk me into carrying on. One by one, the scenes go by. They throw me into school situations and job situations. At my mother's suggestion, I apply for a receptionist's job at a clinic, only to learn to my horror it is a pet clinic. I have never been at ease with animals. I feel as if I am drowning and I find myself admitting that I can't stand to have anything dependent on me. I apologize to the man for taking up his time, but I decline the job and get out of there.

They try me in every situation they can think of until we are growing very tired and the doctor announces we will call it a night. It has been the most exciting night I have spent in over a year. In spite of everything, I feel elated.

At the great central staircase, the student nurse asks me to take part in an experiment. They want to know if someone who has experienced a mental breakdown will be more sensitive to surroundings, if blind, than someone presumed normal. Will I wear a blindfold all the way back to the ward? She will wear one too, and we can compare reactions.

Of course I agree, and our blindfolds are carefully adjusted. I have climbed three or four steps when a young man steps up beside me. "It isn't against the rules to have a guide," he announces. There is something familiar about his voice but I can't place it. He says he has a cold. He sounds to me like someone faking a cold. Cautiously, I make my way up that long staircase, grateful to have someone with me when we reach the top, because I feel very uncertain about the top step.

At the visitors' corridor, the young man leads me to a chair and we sit and chat for a few minutes. He tells me he is a psychologist and I ask if he is going to be on the staff. I am disappointed when he says he won't be. I feel the kind of acceptance from him that is so rare between staff and patients here. I will miss this supportive empathy and I expect to have a depressive reaction when I realize I will never really get a look at him. He walks me to the ward door and gives my shoulder a farewell squeeze. "You are going to get well," he tells me, and I can't help but believe. How I wish he was staying. No one else has been able to make me believe.

I arrive on the ward literally hysterical with some kind of triumph, spilling it all out in a torrent of words to the nurses. Dr. Winchell follows me to the ward and we have a short chat in the conference room. I like and trust Dr. Winchell. He is kind and sympathetic. I am glad I don't have to talk to an analyst tonight. Dr. Winchell is encouraging, calm, and secure. He hands me a scrap of paper on which is written:

> Truth is, in our world, undergoing a terrific battle to maintain its existence. It shines brightly at times but many clouds obscure it. It is being ravished, prostituted, and distorted but it is fighting bravely and the battle ebbs and flows.

So much mental illness is caused because people continue to look into the glass darkly, instead of face-to-face. They want me to see reality. They want me to see truth.

෴

A decade later, I was training in psychiatric nursing in the hospital where I had been a patient. A relief nurse was sent to our unit one night, an old-timer who had nursed me. As we sat talking around the coffee table, she mentioned a thrilling word I hadn't heard in a long time, the word "psychodrama."

"Were you at my psychodrama?" I asked.

"No," she replied, "But I was on the ward when you came back."

I knew from the twinkle in her eye she remembered more than I did about the intensity of that night—the crazy cloud of love and glitter that had me in a whirl. I had been acting, acting, ACTING! I had been acting well enough to please any of my former teachers at the radio academy. It was a little while before the impact of the experience flooded my being and dropped me from the heights. My doctor told me later my acting had caused them to cancel some planned scenes and call a halt to the drama. I was not confronting myself. I was avoiding that by becoming somebody else.

I suppose my failure to break down explains why it took years before the experience became clear for me. Almost everything happened on that assembly hall stage that night: my attitudes to parents and home, job, boss, authority, people, friends of all ages, to culture, religion, life. It was a soul-searching experience, but the mental patient who has the guts to face up a psychodrama will probably have the guts to face up to reality.

When I graduated as a psychiatric nurse, a nice young man at our graduation formal asked me to dance. His name was Dr. Wray and he told me, "The last time I was in this assembly hall, I was in the balcony watching a psychodrama."

I still have the scrap of paper Dr. Winchell handed to me after the psychodrama. It has split at all the folds and the penciled message is fading, but it is a reminder that the truth must continue to battle, for the truth must prevail.

INTERVAL

After I left hospital I went to work as a stenographer at a wholesale grocers, a boring job. I found a light housekeeping room where I really liked my landlady and the other roomers, but I had to fight depression, loneliness, and the threat of suicide. Weyburn was used to having the mentally ill around, so I was well accepted. Balancing my life as to work and hobbies was still a problem. To live "normally" seemed impossible for me. Routine made my sides ache. Women's clubs bored me to tears. I hated cards, drinking parties, and ball games. At the same time, I made friends, joined an art class, and fought the negative feelings for nearly a year, but in the end I quit my job and ran back to my psychiatrist, who had moved to Saskatoon. He refused to see me, insisting

I learn to take responsibility, so I returned to Weyburn. There luck found me. I got a job as a stenographer in a law office where I really liked the people. I was part of a group that started a Little Theatre group in town and was soon directing *Papa Is All*. In 1951 I began to publish stories. I'd been "writing" for years, but I began to work at it seriously.

In the summer of 1951, while working at the law office, I learned that the newly formed Saskatchewan Arts Board was going to hold drama classes at a summer workshop at Fort Qu'Appelle. I arranged for my holidays and was off to take drama from Burton and Florence James. A year later I returned to the workshops to take a writing class from W.O. Mitchell. As a result I was offered a job as assistant executive secretary of the Arts Board. I had misgivings. Weyburn had really become home. Besides, my dad had been discharged from the hospital after all those years and was building a little house by the Souris River, right where the highway entered the city.

But the Arts Board beckoned, and I suppose I felt it was my destiny. I resigned my job at the law office and moved to Regina. It was not all good. I was living with Mother again, a situation so fraught with tension that she finally went to visit a cousin in Indian Head and left a note to tell me she wouldn't come back until I was out of the suite. So I got a suite of my own, but I didn't feel at all at home. I was soon very involved in Regina Little Theatre productions and I found much about my job interesting, but I liked to be *doing* creative projects. I really didn't like promotion. Besides, there was too much uncertainty, too many arbitrary decisions, too much temperament . . . I finally saw a psychiatrist who told me he believed anyone who worked for the Arts Board would go crazy. I took the hint, but, looking back, I wonder at the stupidity of my next decision—I returned to Toronto.

Worst move yet. I took a job in a law office and promptly went spinning down the rabbit hole again. A doctor told me to return to Saskatchewan, but I didn't. I remembered everything I had learned in the mental hospital about rest and diet and hobbies and I simply lived through the breakdown on my own. It took four months and then I was able to go to work for Office Overload. Oddly, the next seven months were among the most interesting in my life. I worked in a wide variety of offices, from engineering to advertising to trucking, and I had time to think and get things into perspective. It provided background for what I really wanted to do with my life— teaching sociology—but that was still far in the future.

When I got the letter telling me of the new superintendent and the improvements happening at the mental hospital, I was intrigued. It began to look as if I was destined to be involved with psychiatry. I returned to

Weyburn and moved in with my father. His little cottage was not modernized, had no running water and no insulation, but I had lived most of my life in uncomfortable conditions so that didn't bother me. I still had friends in town. I spent the winter of 1955–56 writing and weighing the idea of trying for a job at the mental hospital. Did I have the nerve? Would they consider me?

In the spring of 1956 I went back to The Mental in the strange new role of staff. In September I enrolled as a student of psychiatric nursing and set out on a three-year program to learn something concrete about mental illness, to find a new and worthwhile interest in trying to help those who were sick like me.

PSYCHIATRIC NURSE

n the second year of my training period, my wing cap
with rounded corners was brightened by a yellow ribbon
to signify my status as a second-year student psychiatric nurse. Our uniforms were archaic. The basic dress of
medium blue had a fine white stripe, and over it we wore a
bib starched to breastplate texture, a voluminous starched
apron that had to reach a regulation seven inches below
the knee, and a three-inch belt of white cotton starched
to the consistency of iron, over and under which a key
clip was intricately fastened. The "blues" were collared
and cuffed in cotton porcelain, which rubbed the throat
and usually (on my uniform) gaped at the neck. I was
forever parting my apron at the back and giving a tug
to the tails of my bib in an attempt to overcome chronic

gaposis. Our hair was not allowed to touch our collars so I went about with mine shingled and looked bald under my cap. Pinning the collars and cuffs to the blues and pushing the pearl button studs through eyeholes in the belt were the biggest tasks connected with dressing. At first it took me twenty minutes to whip into uniform.

But oh, that hefty belt made one feel small-waisted, protected, and light of foot. The apron swished, the keys rattled, and the caps were breezy. The uniform did all it could to make us feel military and aloof from our patients. That is why, eventually, it went the way of the hospital dome.

Morale can be very low in a mental hospital, but ours was fairly high. Our hands, in many wards where the aged and bedridden lived, were still in urine and feces, and our feet were very much on the ground, often plodding along beside groups of long-term patients who had been stored in the building for so long they had forgotten how to communicate, but our heads were swimming with new ideas. Among us were those who worked only for a paycheque, but their ranks were dwindling. Among us, too, were people of knowledge and professional pride. We were proud of our training, determined to graduate, to win the right to wear the insignia of the registered psychiatric nurse: maroon ties for the men, and for the women two maroon velvet bands.

We were paid to train—minimal wages to start and yearly increases—and in exchange we worked an eight-hour shift on wards. We then attended two hours of lectures each weekday, with homework and study time extra. It was hardest when we were on night shift, for then we had to get up early each afternoon to go to the hospital to attend class, and a shift lasted four weeks. We were permitted a very small margin of absenteeism from ward work or class, and if we exceeded it we could not graduate. Our passing mark was sixty and our passing average was high. This grind continued from September through May, and then we were free from class and merely did our regular work on wards, with a short vacation period. In third year they reduced our workday and allowed us time off for lectures. Third year also included a wonderful month when we were exempt from ward work altogether and spent full days in seminar with nine or ten of our fellow students.

Such a comment suggests that I enjoyed class better than ward work, which may be correct. The challenge of ward work, in a large hospital, depended a great deal on the level of the ward, and though I found it rewarding, I also found it heavy, physically. But I valued the opportunity to learn psychiatry in such a setting, and it was, to my mind, a superior educational experience to the isolated, academic work of university. It was, if we cared to use it so, an intense growing experience. I have never felt closer to a group than I did to the students who went through seminar with me. We were spirited and unified, and it is a month that stands out like a constellation in my memory.

The big mental hospital was an impersonal horror of regimentation and authoritarianism, not to mention noise, crowding, and neglect. It was bureaucratic at its best, inhumane and brutal at its frustrated worst. But it had something that small units will never be able to duplicate unless and until society makes tremendous adjustments in the way it is willing to spend money. The big mental hospital had a nucleus of the professional specialists who are necessary to the best treatment of mental illness, and it had them all there in one place, available, and able to co-ordinate their use of facilities. Our hospital had a professional occupational therapist (OT) with a large staff, all of whom had training in psychiatric nursing, and the OT also supervised a recreational therapist and staff. Music and art therapies supplemented crafts. There was a ward activities program to see that patients who did not participate in regular group activities had access to craft materials, instruction, and recreation right on their wards. The hospital also had a social therapist, whose job was to organize parties and to coordinate the work of visiting volunteers. We had a small bowling alley, an assembly hall with stage, balcony, and motion picture projector, and we had ball diamonds, bowling lawns, tennis courts, skating and curling rinks. We had sports equipment ranging from medicine balls to bikes. To expand our facilities and help in the resocialization of patients, we had arrangements to take patients to a bowling alley, a movie theatre, and a public swimming pool downtown. To try to make up for a relative shortage of psychiatrists and psychologists, a number of our graduate nurses had taken clinical training, and these clinical nursing officers were available for consultation and did psychotherapy with patients.

When I look back at that hospital where I trained, I am ashamed of some of our attitudes. We had a lot to learn about human rights. But when I think of what attitudes had been, what they were still in many hospitals, I know that we had taken giant steps. I recall some of the basics of our training—the kind of things we were taught during our first week of orientation—and they are still the *a b c*'s and *d*'s of psychiatric nursing:

1. A mental breakdown could happen to anyone. The mentally ill are not freaks or inferiors. No one is "immune."

2. A person is a whole—a physio-socio-psychological being—and it is the whole person who must be treated.

3. Every patient is an individual, with individual needs and differences.

4. No case of mental illness should be viewed as hopeless.

These were our foundation stones. On them we were trying to build a therapeutic structure. The big hospital sometimes abetted the process and sometimes blocked it. There were so many polarities: mechanical vs. organic, authoritarian vs. democratic, staff vs. patients. In the old days, staff were guards, protecting the public from the insane and the insane from each other. We were trying to build a treatment situation in which patients and staff were in something together. Our teachers were devoted to helping us to understand. I remember the voice of a male supervisor, speaking to a newly admitted patient, "We'll work together, you and I, and we'll lick this thing." I remember other voices, staff who thought of patients as another breed and referred to them as "them," who would not do so much as put a toe in the new water. Fear of mental illness is the archenemy of the psychiatric nurse.

The real issue, though it was too often covert, was historically based and much broader in scope than just our individual hospital. We often floundered around in our own private arena, worrying about how to make the hospital environment both relaxing and stimulating, and thereby more therapeutic, or worrying about how to make our attitudes more humane. Often the short-sighted individual skirmishes blinded us to the real problem—that the central goal and purpose of our hospital was being drastically changed and too many people were unaware of the shift. The general public had to become oriented to the new purpose, but so did the staff, and, believe it or not, so did the patients. "Mental hospital" still produced mental imagery of "asylum," which had become a synonym for "prison" or "punishment," or, at best, "custodial care." For generations, the public had built these places to rid society of the mentally unstable, to protect society from them at all costs, with no regard for the comfort or well-being of the inmates. Our goal now was to see to the well-being of the patients, and wherever possible to return them to the society that had rejected them. Small wonder hundreds of people were confused. We had pulled a gigantic switcheroo, and though the policy makers were using caution and common sense, we could hardly expect to change centuries-old attitudes overnight.

The chief legacy inherited from the old regime was the value placed upon order. That's what mental hospitals had been about—the control and repression of deviance, the denial by force of any threat to middle-class conformity. Typical of our double dilemma, then, was the confusion between order and tolerance. Our training was weighted heavily in favour of tolerance. We were taught to understand, to question why, to try to put ourselves in the patient's place, to concentrate upon his special needs. To our great frustration, many of the nursing units were weighted heavily in favour of order, and some supervisors judged nurses more for their ability to get through the meals and medications and other routines with alacrity, and less for their ability to relate to patients. But military discipline was fast disappearing. Staff no longer stood to attention when senior nurses or doctors entered the ward. The distance between beds no longer had to be measured, the spreads no longer had to be tight or the corners turned to an exact 45° angle. Everywhere, nurses and patients could be seen working and playing together. Nurses would sit at the breakfast table chatting with the patients over a cup of coffee, although it was rare to see a nurse drinking from the patients' cups. Most would unlock a special cupboard and get a "staff cup" before they would join patients at breakfast. Of such incongruities were our daily lives constructed. The hospital was burdened with rules and regulations, and the smallest transaction required paper work. Every item purchased for or by a patient had to be recorded, every item lost or destroyed had to be checked off. Every sign of problem or of improvement, of course, had to be reported. Countless restraints were supposed to keep the staff in line: no visiting from ward to ward, no reading on night duty, no this, no that. Most of us treated minor regulations with almost boisterous disregard, but major ones, like the twenty-minute meal period, we had to accept. Every ward supervisor differed, and we all knew who was fussy, who severe, and who lax. On some wards you counted the dirty laundry before you went off duty, if you broke your back to do it. On other wards, if emergencies kept you from finishing such tasks, you were allowed to leave them for the oncoming shift. Female supervisors had the reputation of being far more rigid about such regulations than male supervisors. Staff members could be turned in for insubordination and various kinds of rule breaking, but this was rarely done. There was a strong norm against brutality toward patients, and yet there was an even stronger norm against squealing.

Fortunately, we had enough constructive goals to fill up a lot of our time. It taxed our creative initiative to find activities to interest our patients and to motivate our patients to participate. Withdrawal is the chief symptom of schizophrenia, and we confronted it constantly. If we succeeded in getting two usually mute patients with schizophrenia to speak to each other, or even to exchange smiles, it might be greeted as a triumph. Since many of our patients had been ill for years and seemed to have forgotten how to communicate, stimulating communication had high priority. The nurse saw herself as a bridge, over which the patient might be encouraged to pass on a journey from the "other world" in which he had been living back to the "world of reality" where the rest of us were. In order to assist someone to make such a passage, it is essential to establish trust. Our interpersonal relationships with our patients were the key to our success in psychiatric nursing, and they called for understanding, not only of the patient but of ourselves. We learned to keep a searchlight sweeping continually over our inner motivations, as we sought to know our patients.

UNDERSTANDING

While I was in training I kept a journal; much of the material in the chapters that follow is taken from what I wrote there.

I've been told by well-meaning friends that I should stop thinking and learn to do as I'm told, and let the hospital go its own way, because it will anyway. But I am thirty-five years old and I have eighteen years of education and another profession, and it is not easy to take the role of student at all times. When I feel the lack of autonomy too keenly I have to go back and remind myself that I may be a teacher and a law stenographer and the former assistant executive secretary of the Saskatchewan Arts Board, etc., but in psychiatric nursing I am still a novice and that is how it is. I guess the worst of it is being trapped in the bigness of an institution like this.

I've been going through one of my "What-on-earth-am-I-doing-here?" days. I can't imagine how I'm getting away with it. I'm not a nurse. I never wanted to be a nurse. I wanted to be an actress and a writer and an artist, and I wasn't a bad teacher, but I sure never planned to be a nurse. I'm faking it and I know it—*acting* a nurse. The reluctance of some of the old timers to accept me is not so much that I'm an ex-patient and don't fit in; it's because I'm a pseudo and therefore I don't fit in.

I remember what Dr. Rejskind said to me when I joined the staff: "Why do you try so hard to be normal?" But Dr. Rejskind isn't just a psychiatrist, he's a good psychiatrist. The minister at my church questioned me too: "Are you sure you're doing the right thing?" Of course Ann Saddlemeyer said it best. She wrote in haste to say, "Always knew you were a Tom Sawyer, but I never thought you'd go to all that trouble to set a free man free."

Well, yes, I would, and I can't think of a more exciting place to be at this time than Dr. Humphry Osmond's mental hospital. I asked myself if I'd rather be back at CBC, and there was a resounding "No!" Then I asked about the Arts Board and got the same negative response. It was partly to keep from being re-absorbed by the Board that I decided to come on staff as an aide.

I remember how I reacted to the hospital when I began to get well and see things realistically. I thought, "This is *real* drama," and from then on the artificiality of theatre oppressed me. I lost motivation and could get no satisfaction out of it. I had seen real life drama and wanted back in. Well, I'm back in up to my neck and, when I'm having a good day, I simply love it here. It is as if every dream I ever had as a patient is coming true—all kinds of patients participating in sports and arts who were just sitting neglected in those days. Ward activities! I never could see why we couldn't have craft materials right on the wards. Now we have, and instructors, and pianos.

I only wish they'd ditch the TV and radio. The place is noisy enough without radios blaring. Noise is aggravating. When the ancient Greeks treated people by letting them sit in beautiful gardens with music playing, they weren't blaring radios at them—they were playing flutes. There is a difference. Music therapy gives us a taste of that, but it is only for an hour once or twice a week. Not enough. There isn't enough of anything, I guess, but when I watch all that is going on I feel absolutely joyful. Hopeless, but joyful. A paradox. That's The Mental. Would anyone ever be able to put this place into suitable words? Now we are on the verge of bringing sane people into the land of the insane through the use of psychedelic drugs. Breakthrough or false move? Who knows? I don't think there are answers in psychiatry. Only questions, and experimentation, and endless unexplored territory.

One of the most encouraging things that has happened to me here is the discovery that I can talk to people who have had the experience of taking mescalin or lysergic acid, and they will accept the things I tell them about my adventures without asking stupid questions or withdrawing into a safe, smug world of disbelief. So LSD has given me the first hope I've had in a decade that people might actually come to understand, but I'm growing sceptical. How can anyone know, after just a few hours in Underland, what it feels like to be there for years? I've heard no one reporting voices, and voices are the bulk of hallucinations. I guess I should be glad there are brave souls willing to try, even if it is only for eight hours. I'd like to take the drug, just to see if it bears any resemblance to what I experienced ten years ago, but Dr. Osmond has vetoed the idea, "in case I get into a place I can't get out of."

I doubt that. I've got out of some pretty strange places, although visual hallucinations didn't have much to do with it. It was more like getting deep into my mental storage and wandering in endless vaults among dusty cobwebs and dangerous quagmires, with voices promising me wonderful things if I would just keep the faith and hang on. Is that why I have this uneasy feeling that biochemistry may lead psychiatry up a blind alley? I don't mean that they're wrong. I'm sure they're right. It's just that I don't think understanding the brain physically is going to give us all the answers. I found something so creative about the trip through the head—but there I go translating my breakdown as relevant to someone else. I had to take an oral exam from Dr. Rejskind during finals, and he said, "I must warn you never to think you understand another patient based on your own experience. Everyone is different." I know that, but I know my breakdown had spiritual overtones. Of course they talk about LSD being a spiritual experience, but in the meantime Dr. Hoffer is systematically testing urine in a search for abnormalities. I suppose I am the short-sighted one.

Someone asked me recently what treatment I thought benefited me most when I was a patient here, and I said, "Hypnotherapy." Surprised myself, but I remember the vast sense of relief I felt after my one treatment with hypnosis. Dr. Selinger said it would take years to recover and face the traumas that had made me ill and I know it will. They come up bitter as gall, and it takes a lot of strength to face them and work them out. There is such a difference between the muddled emotions I felt when I was ill and the feelings I call real emotions. That may be the real reason I am curious enough to take LSD. Does it lead a person into the personal memories and feelings that are the important aspects of a breakdown, or does it just take you on a sightseeing trip of artistic perceptual constructions?

❧

I've decided to get my old pseudonym out of mothballs and dust if off. I haven't used it since I entered writing contests with it. It may be fun to write an article entitled "Living with Schizophrenia," but I'm not sure I'd want it published under my own name, because I question whether I have schizophrenia. They always said I didn't have what Dad had, manic-depressive psychosis, but my nursing friends are certain I did not have schizophrenia. When I see patients with schizophrenia, I don't see much resemblance to myself, yet I can match them mile for mile with delusions and hallucinations. As Dr. Osmond says, my world was "very fluid." A fluid world is the current criterion for diagnosing schizophrenia. Who am I to disagree with the experts? I rather like the idea that I had schizophrenia and got over it, because MDP frightens me. It is cyclic, and I don't like to think it will keep coming back and hitting me, as if I was tied to a mill wheel and destined to slap the water every time it comes around. But there is something Dr. Osmond does not know. I did have a second breakdown. I had a dilly of a second breakdown, all alone in Toronto in 1954. If I have MDP, I should be due for another one in six years, or soon thereafter. If it happens, I suppose I will have to face it. Meanwhile, my article is to be entitled "Living with Schizophrenia." Makes me wonder how much psychiatric literature we can really trust.

I admire Dr. Osmond so much. He is so bubbly and interesting and intelligent and kind, and so concerned with treating the mentally ill like deserving human beings. He calls schizophrenia an "affront" and he is right. It is such a destructive thing. At the same time, I know he recognizes the creative side. I guess what I am asking is "What is 'well'?" What if a new magic cure takes away the visions and the voices? Will it constitute some kind of loss for mankind? To see the majority of our patients on the long-term wards, it's a wonder I even dare ask.

All of the patients in my group are on Largactil (chlorpromazine hydrochloride). Some are on a holding dose of 50 mg. four times a day and the others are on 25 mg. four times a day. The effect is to make them just a little dopey and slow. I often wondered about that. My friend Linda stole some Largactil from her ward and deliberately took it for four days to see what kind of effect it had. She was convinced that it was stupefying patients without having any beneficial effect at all, and she begged me to try the experiment. I think she thought that because I have had a breakdown, I would be able to tell her if I felt I could have got well under the influence of Largactil. Reluctantly, I let her persuade me, but I never finished the four days. In fact I took four 25 mg. doses on day one and that was that. My report to Linda was that I felt as if someone had placed a heavy granite boulder on my forehead and the entire thinking part of my brain was numbed. I thought of the speeded-up thoughts that had raced through my head during my breakdown, often leading me into dead ends but eventually bringing me through to awareness and insight. I began to feel sick about giving patients Largactil, but I also knew what the ward environment would be like without it. Linda had not lived on the admitting ward next door in the forties. I had. I could still hear the din of a dozen or more disturbed patients screaming in the night. I could remember a time when many of these patients were completely unapproachable. Now they were, to use the jargon, "amenable to therapy." Somebody was robbing Peter to pay Paul, but I couldn't see any alternative. At least we weren't using straight jackets.

∾

Staff solidarity is probably uppermost in a hospital of this kind, where the spectre of violence haunts the background and where every staff member asks himself, "Will the nurses I'm working with tonight stand by if there's any trouble?" To reassure your fellow staff and thereby win acceptance, it is necessary to prove yourself time and time again. You stand by in a fight, voice the right attitudes, and maintain distance from patients to indicate that the "sane" are by some mystic endowment several social notches above the patients. You prove yourself by maintaining discipline and control on your unit. Unless patients jump to do a task when you speak, you are weak, joining with the patients and letting the staff down. If there is undue freedom on your ward, you are suspect.

It's a sad reality, though, that few of the staff realize what it feels like to be on the bottom. They may have lost a playground fight as kids, but that isn't the same as being a patient in a totalitarian camp. There is no escape; no hope that teacher will come out and call off the kids, because teacher is the one who ordered the fight, may even be leading it. That is the mental hospital situation.

I cannot in good conscience maintain social distance between my patients and myself, and I refuse to force them to work on command. Perhaps, then, I overemphasize loyalty to other staff ideals. Perhaps I am unconsciously dedicated to keeping the emotional pot from boiling, kidding myself that a quiet, cooperative patient is a healthy patient.

The road that leads to competence in psychiatric nursing is long and hazardous and, when I look back, I quake to think how hazardous. I have had twenty months of training, fourteen of them with regular lectures, and yet my ignorance is incredible. I have a piece of information here, a bit of advice there, and considerable theory, but I have not had time to get it into perspective. I think I had too thorough a grounding in too many professions before I entered this one. It is a drawback for me, for instance, that I cannot reprimand a patient in front of others, unless it can be done jokingly, or else when the situation is so obvious that it just has to be done. I remember how it was drilled into us at Normal School never to humiliate a student in front of the class, or you would lose his love and loyalty forever and make no progress with him at all. In my drama training, the same thing came up: never jump an actor in front of the rest of the cast, or, again, you have humiliated and harmed him.

We had a sociologist here a while ago who saw the staff as an army fighting a disease known as mental illness, and we talked about it in class. Most of us offered a good deal of resistance to the idea. I think a mental hospital is a school, not a battleground. We are not fighting a disease, we are trying to overcome ignorance and fear. Then isn't my Normal School training the proper course? We are trying to promote happiness by promoting skills in work and hobbies and social life. Then isn't my drama training the proper course? Here again, I feel that my views differ from those of many of the staff that I talk to and listen to. But I believe that if a nurse has the right attitudes her patients can weather a lot of mistakes. I only wish I had paid more attention to one of the most important statements to be heard throughout my psychiatric nursing training: *"We all do the best we can."* That should be the golden rule for understanding others, but it is difficult to grasp.

છ

I have met several of the university students on summer relief, and one of the boys asked me today what prompted me to enter psychiatric nursing. To my own surprise, I found myself telling him about the day I told my doctor I felt guilty because the government was paying for my keep in hospital. I came of a culture where you paid your own way. Now that I was faced with the reality, I didn't feel right about it.

The doctor told me it would be stupid of any government to let people go on being sick, because we need people who can be useful. If they gave me treatment now, in the future I could be a productive member of society too. I felt a great sense of relief, because I knew what it meant to be saddled with a lifetime of worry because you couldn't pay for the care of someone in this hospital. Most of my life, my mother had worried over Dad being here.

My doctor's explanation must have really adhered because, when that boy asked me the question today, I almost said, "I'm paying my debt to society." That is ridiculous. I wasn't a criminal: I was ill. But, like the doctor predicted, I am productive now and I can at least contribute a few years of time and effort to pay back for the nine months spent on me.

KLECKNER

This story isn't about Kleckner, any more than *The Hurricane* was about a hurricane. When Nordoff and Hall wrote *The Hurricane* they wrote about a people and a way of life, and the effect of a catastrophic crisis upon human lives. This is Kleckner's role in this story, for in a mental hospital there are some human beings who can precipitate as much of a crisis as any hurricane. A quick turn of events can mean the difference in the social climate of an entire ward for days, affecting the lives of the hundred patients crowded there.

Our hospital had become a relatively quiet place. It might have been due to tranquilizers, but we liked to think it stemmed from improved environmental conditions and the attitudes of well-trained staff. But it was still an institution for the emotionally disturbed, and seclusion rooms still came into use on refractory wards when a patient went "up the pole" and needed to be isolated from the group for his own sake or for the sake of his fellow patients. We gave the rooms used for this the colloquial name of "side rooms." On some wards we would work for weeks and encounter no disturbances that couldn't be calmed by a little attention and understanding. Where patients are respected as individuals and their quarrels can find a ready mediator, much cause for violence is removed. But we did have our hurricanes, and Kleckner was not the least of these.

For many years local folklore had persisted with a story that the most dangerous patients in the hospital were those with the misfortune to have epilepsy as well as their psychosis, and the belief was well substantiated by experience. We had a small handful of epileptic patients whose periodic disturbances had often menaced the staff. Foremost in this small but awesome group stood Kleckner.

Kleckner was of less than medium height but he was a husky man, with a bull neck and powerful shoulders. He was subject to sudden moods of jealousy, suspicion, and rage. Though he had the intelligence to understand his problems, a lifetime of emotional maladjustment had rendered him unable to keep his temper under control. A sunny man with a sunny smile as long as nothing stood in his way, even at his best he had little frustration tolerance. When he wanted to go outside he wanted to go outside, and it went better for staff who stood ready with the key. When he wanted beer, he went downtown to the beer parlour, thoughtlessly running the risk of being reported and brought back under escort. And when he wanted milk for breakfast he wanted milk for breakfast.

Such a small disappointment roused the hurricane. There was no milk on the breakfast table. The farm delivery was late. It didn't occur to Kleckner to accept the absence of the milk. Instead he threw his dishes off the table and stormed from the dining hall, kicking at chairs and door frames as he went. Had he been able to make more than a few guttural sounds, his language would have been powerful. Staff and patients wisely gave him room, but three male staff followed him along his frantic route back to the ward. Once there, he stormed into the dayroom, threw around a few chairs, and then armed himself with the lids of two ashcans, sharp-edged rounds of stainless steel, about the size of cymbals. A patient with schizophrenia, too ill to realize the danger, stood giggling stupidly right in his path. Kleckner raised the weapon in his right hand.

Our five male staff rushed him then. A patient in a furor can fight several men. My female colleague was on the ward, but all she could do was run to the adjoining ward for reinforcements. At last Kleckner was overpowered and dragged into a side room. The sounds he made were like the roars of a wild beast. His eyes were inhuman. His dark brown hair, so neatly combed when he was well, was in disorder. His clothing was torn. They cuffed him hand and foot, left him a mattress to lie on, and covered him with a blanket.

When I returned from the dining room, I observed through the peephole while the men went in to give him an injection, in case I had to run for more reinforcements. I was a little afraid he would cast off the cuffs and break down the door. It was very strong, but so was Kleckner. They gave him heavy sedation, but it took no effect. Kleckner was away to a long disturbance.

When the staff had time to count casualties, they found scraped shins, bruises, and a quantity of scratches. Two of the boys had lost skin from their faces and were rushed to the sick ward for penicillin shots. They came back brilliantly painted with merthiolate and were battle-scarred conversation pieces for days. They teased my colleague and me for running away from a fight, but they didn't minimize the danger. They suggested that female staff stay out of the dayroom unless there were several male staff present, and not wander the ward too much alone.

"It's a kind of climate," the assistant supervisor explained. "A thing like this touches off a lot of excitement sometimes."

There was tension in the air all day and we felt uneasy when we took our groups to occupational therapy, wondering what was happening back on the ward. Kleckner's noises were still fierce, his eyes still wild. A senior nursing officer decided the staff had neglected psychotherapy in the case, so he entered the side room to have a talk with the patient. Handcuffs and all, Kleckner gave him a brutal blow in the face. I was surprised to learn that some of my colleagues shared my sense of threat. It was as if that heavy oak door wasn't even there.

On the second day the episode began to tell on our nerves. The story was repeated, full of colour. The men placed a guard on the door when they took in his breakfast tray. They were no cowards but Kleckner was tough. Unless you had seen that face and heard those sounds, you couldn't imagine how tough.

"But he's a human being," they said. "They're all human beings. Today you'd wonder."

No word of blame for his behaviour. No show of brutality toward him. Just wariness. Male psychiatric nurses seem to come in two categories: either the worst nurses possible, surpassing the laziest of women, or nurses who take their work in stride with a skill and ease beyond the capacity of any woman. I have sometimes been over-whelmed by their great tolerance.

Our ward aide sustained severe scratches to the back of his hand when he took in the tray. "If you lose any more skin you'll start to contract," they laughed.

It's the way you have to take things at the mental hospital. It's unwise to park your sense of humour on the shelf at such a time. But the aide was spending his first summer in a mental hospital and he was quite shaken. He was a college student, usually a good sport, an enthusiastic leader of patient activities and a beaver for work. His reaction to Kleckner's episode surprised us. He became so silent he was almost sullen. He went about with his eyes downcast and a depressed droop to his shoulders. We girls worried about him a little, but then we began to worry about ourselves.

During the first day of the storm a few remarks had been made concerning our safety. On the second day it transpired that our presence on the ward was felt to be unfair to the male staff. They still expected further disturbances, like a chain reaction, to be touched off by the explosion, and women would be more than useless. The men felt they would have to protect us, as well as the patients. The staff situation really was inadequate—the five male graduates booked to our shift were never on duty simultaneously, and we were about to enter a four-day stretch when days off would reduce the graduate staff to three. Of these, two were older men not in the peak of health, who should not be expected to fight. We heard that the male staff had decided to approach the supervisor and see if we could be temporarily exchanged for men. We locked ourselves up in the washroom and held a conference.

"They're cooking it up," my colleague said decidedly. "They're not cowards and they're not helpless. They'd get floats in an emergency whether we were here or not."

"We'd look like quitters," I said.

"Women have worked this ward for ten months and never asked off."

"We're not asking off. We're liable to be shoved off."

"To ninety percent of the staff, we'd be asking off. They all know about Kleckner, but they wouldn't have any way of knowing the rest of the story."

"They're using smart psychology. Making it look as if they want to be rid of us. Hard to know if they mean it or not."

"Neat," she agreed. "Let's be selfish about it."

"Game," I said. "We may not get away with it, but the least we can do is refuse to go."

Our pact came to nothing, because the supervisor laughed when they approached him about our transfer. He had handled his ward for several years and it would be kept under control without exchanging staff. The women would stay. We were relieved and the men ceased to talk about it, except for the ward aid.

On the third afternoon they took Kleckner out of the side room for the first time, and three men walked him to the patients' washroom for a cleanup. He was subdued, but they carried a sheet to immobilize him should he decide to break loose. We girls locked ourselves in the office and stayed beside the phone until they gave us the all-clear. We discussed the possibility that we had been too selfish. The ward was noisier, more quarrelsome. You could feel the static snapping in the air. When I approached my group to come to their activities, I never knew if they would smile back at me or strike. I felt as if I was walking a tightrope over the snake pit, beginning to wonder if I would come to the end of it.

Every member of my group had been hospitalized more than ten years and they had all given up verbal communication except one. He spoke in response to questions but seldom initiated conversation. They made the sort of group that is an almost insurmountable challenge to a nurse. They were strange, repressed personalities, full of lost hope, although the supervisor encouraged me by telling me how much they had improved after two years of group therapy.

"It's just that you can't see it in a few weeks," he explained. "The change is slow, but I've seen them come a long way since we started the group. Some of these fellows used to be full-time side room patients. It takes time."

And I was being paid to give them a month of time. So we plugged ahead, making our beds, pitching and catching our medicine ball, smoking our cigarettes, cutting with our fretsaws, colouring with our crayons, going for walks and ballgames, and having our thrice-weekly shaves. Plugging along. Trying to establish a bit of trust in someone who had lost faith in all humanity. Trying to get a guy to speak whose illness had made him withdraw from conversation for fifteen years. We might be rewarded by a friendly smile of recognition on a still youthful face, a gesture of politeness once in three weeks, a spark of interest when they heard a story from *Reader's Digest* about a man who carved portraits of rock in the Black Hills. Getting guys who had paid no attention to their fellow human beings for years to toss a ball back and forth with a bit of laughter, or to sit together and play instruments in a rhythm band— all this was reward. It was worth entering the dismal grey cement basement where the male refractory ward was entombed. It was worth the danger. It was worth the ever-present threat of Kleckner, living out his furor behind that locked door.

On the fourth morning, following breakfast, I went as usual to the side room off the dayroom where my group slept, and began to make beds. Two of my six patients could make their own beds with persuasion, but I usually had to make the other four. The ward aide stepped in to help me. He didn't really have time, because the boys scrubbed the entire dayroom and corridor each morning, but evidently he wanted to talk. He was still worried about the girls. He couldn't understand the attitude of the supervisor or accept that a man would submit women to such a vulgar atmosphere and to such danger.

"It's not as if you were toughs," he said. "You weren't spawned on the waterfront. You're intelligent, educated young women training to be psychiatric nurses. It's blind and cruel. I don't get this business of booking female staff to male wards anyway. Especially a ward like this. What's the hospital trying to prove? That everything's so well under control that women can work on the worst ward in the place?"

He made it sound as if we were working under a dictatorship and lacked the sense to strike against it. In his first-season insecurity, he was belittling everything we were doing, and it made me angry.

"Do you think the ward would be any different if we weren't here?" I asked bluntly.

He paused. "No," he lied. Then he corrected himself. "Maybe."

"Then we must contribute something to it."

"I think you contribute a lot. You make it more pleasant to work here, more fun, something to look forward to. You have an effect on the language we use, the way we treat the patients. You can't help but have an effect."

"But do we contribute anything to the patients?"

"Indirectly. By having an effect on staff. It's bound to affect the patients."

"But not directly?" I persisted, burning with resentment. I had tried to give energy and interest to my group, yet I was aware of a sense of guilt that my interest was less and my energy slack compared to what I had used on other units. In the face of doubts, this verbal blasting of our work infuriated me. But I liked and respected the young aide, and I wanted to get across to him the vaguely formed reason I had for being there. It had something to do with the contrast between the dorm we were in and me. Often I had felt that contrast—the funny feeling of being entirely out of place somewhere, of being alien and looking foolish. It was always intensified in the group dorms. The walls and floors were brick and cement, though in the small rooms walls were now brightly painted. The beds were low narrow cots made up with white spreads, stark and lonely. The ward smelled of sweat and urine and the myriad odours of untidy human beings. The words I could hear if I listened were often the last word in profanity. In the midst of it, dressed in white apron over my student blues, with a cap on my curly hair and lipstick on my mouth, I sometimes felt rather fragile and beautiful, like a flower in the midst of the desert, and every bit as likely to wilt and die unseen. Yet always on the tail of this alien feeling came the other feeling: "I am here for a purpose. This is not for nothing. I must have some influence here."

The new aide, uncertain of purpose and without benefit of any training, had pricked my sacred bubble. I looked at his rakishly scarred face and fought back the tears.

"I hope your attitude doesn't reflect the general attitude of the male staff," I said, "or we've been kidding ourselves that we do any good here. What does a woman contribute to a home?"

"She makes a home!" he said. "She gives it gentleness."

"Maybe we can't do it here," I said. "Maybe we are wasting our time. But we can try. These guys have seen hate and cruelty and ugliness. Can we do any harm by trying to show them something else?"

"I haven't been here long enough to give me the right to talk," he admitted. "I should dry up. But from what the others say, female staff have made a huge difference to the male side, especially here. I was just worked up. I wouldn't want to see my mother or my sister down here while Kleckner was in a state like this."

"I'm a bad example," I said, still feeling sorry for myself. "I was raised without men in my home and I don't know much about handling them. Perhaps another woman would show better results."

"You do great," he assured me, tucking in a bedspread nervously. I could see that he was experiencing not so much a change of tune as a gradual evolution of thought. "Both of you. You do contribute to the ward—a lot. But is it valuable to you as part of your training? These fellows are so slow about relating to anybody, especially women. I wonder if it would be better if graduate nurses came down."

"It is a kind of valley in my training," I said, realizing that the slow pace of the ward had been frustrating. "But it will be valuable for that very reason. You have to learn to change your pace. If you can't relate to patients who don't talk, you don't make much of a psychiatric nurse."

"I still don't see why you were stubborn about getting off. A crisis is a crisis. Whole armies have to retreat at times."

I hate the misused military metaphor in connection with a mental hospital, so I said flatly, "We are no army."

"What if the new program were held up a day or two? A week? If it was held up ten years or a century, we'd finally get there. Things develop. Why did you make an issue of staying here through this?"

It suddenly filtered into my mind that he was actually concerned about us as people, but I was thinking of something else. We had almost finished the last bed and the dorm looked bright and tidy. A line from a play came out of memory and repeated itself several times. It was a line from *The Corn Is Green*, ". . . if a light should come into the mine." That was all.

"Then somebody else could fight our battle over again," I said, "and either win or ask off, as you wanted us to do."

"It isn't really this situation we're discussing," he said. "It's a principle."

"Of course it's a principle. If you lose courage once, it's hard to get it back. We've always got to hold the ground we've won."

"It's not that principle," he said. "Aren't you trying to prove that you're as good as the men?"

I anticipated the thrust and smiled. "Don't be an idiot," I said. "We haven't the strength or the power of men, and we could never take control of a ward like this the way they do. If I want to prove anything it's simply that women are needed here and that we have a role here, just as the men do. It's not better. It's different, and it isn't formed yet. Maybe that's the real problem."

"I feel a bit differently about it," he said. "I'm glad I talked to you."

"You know my father used to be a patient here," I said, as he paused at the door. "It will help you to understand if I tell you something else. My father lived for years on this very ward."

I could see in the look of sympathy that came to his eyes that the boy was going to give up psychiatry. It takes a certain kind of stomach, and his was going to turn.

I didn't tell him that, just a few days earlier, I had asked Dad why he had never asked for transfer to a better unit. After all, he was a trustee. Dad replied, "I liked it there. They didn't interfere as much!" Apparently, as an old-timer who'd learned to live a private life in the midst of madness, Dad failed to appreciate attempts at psychotherapy. I wondered what he would think of the basement ward now.

The next room was always a shambles because one of its occupants sat on his bed all day spitting tobacco juice. I changed his spread, turned the corners, pulled it tight. Then I noticed that someone had stripped Kleckner's unused bed and laid out a pile of fresh folded linen on the bare mattress. I pushed the bed from the wall and got behind it, starting to lay out the bottom sheet. There was a movement on the other side of the bed and I looked up. There, big as life and properly dressed, was Kleckner.

I tried not to react. Should I slide out quietly and unobtrusively or stand my ground? Then Kleckner smiled and gestured that he intended to make the other side of the bed. I smiled back. My heart went down to its proper place again. He was okay. They must have let him out. Kleckner in control of himself is childish and selfish, but he is not a threat to life and limb. He is very different from the other Kleckner. That afternoon they reissued his parole and let him go outside. It is better to reward his good behaviour than to punish him for what is beyond his control. Kleckner will go on and on, through storm after storm, and whether there will ever be much change in a personality long warped and distorted in so many ways is improbable. But as I said at the beginning, this story isn't about Kleckner.

AN AFTERNOON IN THE SUN

I remember feeling apprehensive as I approached the bulletin board where our new assignments were posted. I had already been on female admissions and on recreation, the female "sick ward," a male continued treatment ward where I led my first group, and even male refractory. (Had anyone told me when I applied to work at the hospital that I would be expected to work on male refractory, even for a month, I might not have had the nerve to try. But it proved to be a fairly satisfying experience, if only because it laid to rest the shapeless fears that most of us carried about unseen corners of the hospital.) This time I was going to a good ward, a female continued-treatment unit housing 110 patients, where the average level of interaction was fair to good. The ward was organized to meet challenges and reduce apathy. Thought had gone into choosing the right activities for the right patient, and there was no such thing as a forgotten patient. Every patient had a nurse, every day, and patients who rejected all our invitations to participate were always there, in the backs of our minds, as we tried to think of something to interest them, something to bring them back to the social group.

The group therapy on the ward was similar to that being used throughout the hospital, and I confess I found it short of inspirational. When group therapy first appeared in our hospital, ten years earlier, it was seen as a shortcut to psychotherapy, enabling one psychologist to reach a number of patients at one time, while at the same time taking advantage of the social milieu of the group. As it spread through the hospital it deteriorated, at least in my opinion. I felt the individual patient had been lost in the group and that many staff believed groups existed to develop conformity and co-operation on the part of the members. However, better to be in a group than to be a forgotten or neglected patient, I told myself, as I watched little knots of men or women sheepishly following their nurses from activity to activity. But was it therapy? Should it be called expediency? Our instructors, who were some of the greatest people I have ever known, refused to look on the darker side. Instead, they taught us where to find chinks of light. They encouraged, they explained the long years of patience required to coach a non-responsive patient back to society, they gave suggestions, they made comparisons with the bad old days, and they struck a persistent note of optimism. They patted us on the back and sent us out to fish in the slough of despond, and even made us believe that one day we might catch something valuable

I was pleased to find that I was booked to lead a group on my new ward. Our group timetable was varied and it left us a little free time. There was usually an hour in the afternoon when we could take a walk or make a visit to the canteen, so my group of seven had lots of opportunity for spontaneous activities.

෩

I've been looking back over my first weeks on the ward, and, as far as I'm concerned, the low point is the Tuesday library period. Although it's booked as library, it's actually a work period. The Recreation office is just off the library, and we are scheduled to clean and tidy both office and library each week. My group has a bad reputation for disliking work, I admit, and there is a feeling in some parts of the institution that they should be doing something for their keep, but I feel that whoever arranged for them to clean the library used poor judgment. They are all intelligent girls, well enough to read and interested in reading, and I get the feeling that going to a library as cleaning women is confusing and even insulting to them. It is like asking a hockey player, just because he is too sick to play, to sweep the ice. I could be wrong, but I know that only Theresa and Laura will cooperate, and they are reluctant. Patsy headed straight for books or comics and curled up on the couch and refused to budge, and Ivy and Joyce did exactly the same. Ruth and Zoe wouldn't go to the library at all, but announced their intention of reading on the ward instead.

The Recreation Department has given me the distinct impression that this lethargy is my fault, because I am obviously not enthused with the project, but I note that in the total five weeks I have led this group they have never bothered to greet us or to tell us what they want us to do. I consider it a wasted hour, and I believe that the group members will never learn to like work by having what appears to be unnecessary tasks thrust upon them, and in a library.

A terrible responsibility rests with the group leader, when you come to think of it. I am mother figure if they have to be washed and combed and fed; leader, friend, helper, or anything you can name. I have to keep a check on their clothing and property, see that they receive medications, and guide their individual and group progress.

It takes a great deal of time, and when staff shortages mean that you must dash to your group five minutes before an activity and round them up, it is hard to make an adjustment. I would hardly expect them to accept a group leader who pays little attention to them.

At noon hour, Patsy, Laura, and Theresa went back to their jigsaw puzzle, which seems to be an ideal drawing card to entice people onto the group veranda. The three were willing to leave the puzzle and come for a walk, and Joyce joined us, but Ruth said she was so scared that her heart was beating so hard it hurt her side. I felt sorry for her, wondering what might be causing the panic, but could give no help. Ivy had her appointment with Mr. Watkin, and of course Zoe won't come outside.

Since the majority of us are fast walkers, we told Joyce we weren't going to take time waiting for her, she could very well keep up with us, and keep up with us she did. We had a marvellous time. First we jumped a mud hole, and then we saw some dark birds with bright yellow tips to their tails that nobody could identify. We studied trees and found a tiny elm only a foot high. We found a culvert and looked through it, bemoaning the fact that we weren't in old slacks so we could crawl through, as we did when we were small. Joyce enjoyed that very much, and had her head into the culvert, peering through. She said it was so much nicer to be outside than in "that place." We cut across the prairie beyond the hospital grounds, and it was wonderful. Real freedom, with the smell of prairie grass and a nice cool breeze. We found a huge old rubber glove some lineman had used for repairing wires, that had a badly burned thumb. Joyce found it, and laughed over it because it was so big. I persuaded her to throw it away again. We found wild roses and mustard and a ball diamond, and I had to explain which of the three schools we could see was which. We passed a new house on the way back, and there was a lot of comment on that. We re-entered the grounds by the footpath beside the hospital ballpark, and Laura's curious eye saw some puffballs. We stopped and discussed those, questioning whether or not they were edible, and Theresa proved to be the best versed in mushroom lore.

"They're all right to eat when they're fresh, early in the morning," she said, "But not when they turn brown. Don't ever eat a brown puffball."

"Don't ever eat a brown puffball," repeated Patsy automatically. She sounded like a five-year-old who, busy learning the world, repeats her new information so she won't forget.

Sometimes I marvel at how enlightened our forebears were to realize how these spreading acres and all the trees along a river would benefit the mentally ill. This is what the Greeks knew. I think they were away ahead of us. I could feel the therapeutic atmosphere all through our walk today.

I didn't talk to the girls about the healthy aspects of our outing, but I didn't have to. You could see it in their faces and hear it in their voices. They were all worlds better after that happy time with nature.

We reached our lawn at ten minutes to two and sat down to relax. Theresa hunted for four-leaf clovers. There was a lot of very friendly small talk. Laura sat with me and told me a tale about what had transpired on my day off. Apparently there was no staff to take the group for a walk, and Mrs. Kearnan suggested to Laura that she take them. Laura refused, saying it was too much responsibility. I noticed that Dianne Fritzke and the independent group were outside, apparently planning to take a walk out the main road to the highway, and I realized Laura was doing some thinking. She indicated Dianne and said, "She mustn't mind responsibility. A person would have to be very reliable to take charge of a group."

"One of these times you should be ready to go on an independent group," I said casually, "like Dianne Fritzke."

"I don't know. When I think of going out without a nurse, it scares me."

"If you were ever to leave hospital you couldn't have a nurse around to look after you. An independent group would be a nice easy step in that direction."

"I couldn't. I'd be afraid."

I was actually afraid, casual as I had tried to sound, that Laura would panic. She was really insecure about such an idea, and, since this was Musical Festival day, I was particularly anxious not to frighten her.

"You take far more responsibility than you realize in this group," I said.

She argued a bit that she did not, because she hates to think that we might convince her that she is better than she wants to be. So we dropped the subject.

When I asked Theresa, equally informally, if she felt that some day she could get along very well in an independent group, there was no anxiety displayed to speak of, except perhaps a slight frown which is very common on her worried little face.

The festival was to begin at 3:15, as soon as the afternoon staff had time to get organized, but I had promised Laura that she would have time to dress and to practice her number before I left, so at 2:20 I told the girls we would have to go in. Laura scarcely repressed a grin, and suddenly I realized that she still intended to beg off. What's more, she knew that I knew.

I made no comment until we were on the ward, and then she beat me to the game. "I have a headache," she said, without preliminary.

"I'll get you an aspirin," I replied quickly, in exactly the same tone of voice.

A rather humorous war of wills ensued, with Laura starting on a tack that would eventually lead to a kind of disintegration of ego, when she would really be unable to make the smallest decision or carry out any preparation. It's a defence mechanism known as disorganization, and Laura knows how to use it. I was ready for it. I went to Laura's locker and made her decisions for her, because we had no time and no strength to withstand a prolonged period of indecision. She began to fuss about what she would wear, and I just picked her pretty flowered silk dress, a bright orange and yellow and white, because it was the one she seemed to be attracted to first, and her white pumps. I refused to listen to her trying to change her mind, I just issued orders. I was glad that I had taken such positive action, because one of our other performers took a fit of stage fright and burrowed into her bed and said she would not sing in the choral group. The two staff who were helping get everyone ready for the festival had eight other patients to encourage, see that they dressed up, see that they had their programs and program numbers, and so forth. The ward was in an uproar.

In the midst of it all, Laura emerged as pretty as a picture, with her hair combed and her makeup nicely applied, and went off to the festival clutching her familiar music book, with a touch of determination in her jaw. I promised to be there to hear her, and I was. I was officially off duty, but I went to the music festival and sat with Theresa and Zoe. To our pride, Laura ended up being just about the best item in the show. She played a waltz. I think the success will give her confidence a boost.

Altogether, I am happy about today. I suppose that is chiefly because of our spontaneous nature walk, which reminded me of how we used to find our own recreation when I was a child on the farm. I think half the trouble here is that everything is so organized; not only bedtime and mealtime and doctor time and meeting time and OT time, but even recreational time. If only we had more room for accidental therapies.

COMMUNITY

eading a group on a high-level continued-treatment ward felt good—there was so much thinking to do. Not that my life was lacking in stimulation. Due to my education and unique psychiatric experiences, I was getting the chance to participate in some of the most interesting intellectual life in the hospital. Dr. Osmond himself was giving me guidance with my writing. I had made a friend in the research department, Gwyn Witney. Aside from the fact that she was full of ideas and compatible, having a pal strategically placed in research had a good side. Most of the staff got the news from the hospital grapevine, and gossip is always distorted as it is passed along. If any department in the hospital really knew what Dr. Osmond and his colleague in Saskatoon,

Dr. Abram Hoffer, were doing or planning to do, it was the research department. It gave me a secure feeling.

The intellectual side of my nursing experience reached its zenith about the time I met the group, and that added another dimension. It began the day my classmate Len Keith beckoned me to his table in the staff dining room to introduce me to a young social anthropologist who had attended their ward meeting that morning. His name was Francis Huxley and he had an English face, blue English eyes, and a clipped English accent.

I asked, "Not one of *the* Huxleys?"

Yes, he was the son of Sir Julian Huxley and the nephew of Aldous. (His father had been knighted that week.)

I blurted, "I once threw your uncle's book across a room and hit the wall with it."

I was aghast that I should have said anything so rude, but he took it well. He asked, "Which book was that?"

"*Brave New World.*"

"He'd be flattered. He didn't expect anybody to take him seriously."

I knew that Dr. Osmond had gone to California and given LSD to Aldous Huxley, but the fact that the illustrious family now had a representative in Weyburn was overwhelming. When I was back on the ward I went up to the first graduate nurse I found and told her excitedly, "There's a Huxley right here in our hospital!"

She looked at me blankly and asked, "What's a huxley?"

Oh well, Weyburn is in the provinces, after all. Francis was to spend several months studying the social interaction patterns of the hospital as they related to the physical layout of the wards, and I soon learned that he had classified me as someone worth getting to know. On my next day off he appeared at my door, asking if I'd like to go for a walk. He was in a mildly pessimistic mood, trying to convince me that hope for world peace is slim and we are likely to have a lot of little atomic bombs dropped on us within the next few decades.

I said, "If that's true, what's the point of doing anything? Why try to help patients? Why write books?"

Francis said, "To write them."

I think that is what it is about Weyburn, these days. It is a place and time when we write them. We get things done and if, in the long run, it is all wiped out, at least we did it.

When we got downtown that day, we bought fresh strawberries and took them with us to the cafe, where we had them with our tea. While we were eating the strawberries, I tried to tell Francis about this feeling I have of being so close to the centre of something; yet I know I'm only a student nurse here, so I'm not likely to get much closer. I said, "It's frightening, because sometimes I feel as if I'm suddenly on a mountain top. What happens after you find yourself on a mountain top? Where do you go from there?"

Francis said, "I guess you climb another mountain top."

Gwyn shares my reaction. The other day she suddenly exulted, "We're here! At the center of the universe! We're where it's all happening!" Much as I love classes and all I'm learning, it worries me that I may be buried alive on a back ward after graduation, and just be there year after year. It is not a future that appeals to me, and yet I can't seem to focus my mind on alternatives.

I had a big argument with Gerry last night (one of the university students spending the summer here). He maintained the hospital was not a community, and I insisted it was. He was using sociology to prove his point: a community is composed of families, people earn their living there, it has to contain three generations, and so on. So we are not a community from that point of view, but surely there are other definitions of community. The word stems from "communication" after all, and the communication here is intense. There is the depth of awareness that comes when people live together in close proximity for decades. Of course, Gerry hasn't been here long enough to pick up on that. No doubt he sees what most people see when they first experience the hospital: hundreds of people who don't communicate at all. Among those who do, a sizeable number don't say anything that can be interpreted by anyone else. Emotional reactions aren't normal. You can't trust many people much of the time.

So why do I maintain this is a community? A friend of mine was in charge of a basement ward one night where she didn't know a single patient. One woman ran a high fever and my friend was asking her name so she could phone head office and report, but the patient was mute and wouldn't or couldn't say who she was. The woman in the cot next to hers was not one to communicate either, but she recognized a crisis and came to the rescue. She said, "Her name is Rena." That was all, but it was enough to let the nurse find the patient's file and arrange to have her taken to the hospital unit.

I remember another story. One of the male staff was watching a football game on TV, along with a number of patients on his ward. He was called out of the dayroom to handle some problem, and when he came back, he asked the score. All was silent. There wasn't a communicative patient in the room at the time. Sensing the need, a usually mute patient with schizophrenia turned his head and told him the score. Nothing more. Why waste words?

There are things Gerry hasn't caught on to yet—how communication zings along beneath the surface in this hospital. These mute patients do sense those around them and they do know what is going on. In fact, one of our instructors, speaking of such patients, warned us, "Watch out what you say in front of a catatonic. Some day he'll write a book and quote you."

There is communication here, day and night. The hospital *is* a community.

NIGHT OF THE RED RUG

Francis Huxley is playing host. He's house-sitting for Dr. Osmond and his family while they are away, and he's probably finding it lonely after senior quarters, so it doesn't strike me as odd that he says, "Come as soon as you've had supper." We work shifts at the mental hospital, so the hours of our social life are a bit erratic. Francis just says, "To hear some music," and it doesn't strike me as odd, either, that he wants to know if I'm working tomorrow. The fact is, I'm facing a double, which means I have the next two days off, so if it turns out to be a late evening, it won't matter.

I'm living with my Dad right across from the hospital grounds where the river road meets the highway into Weyburn, so I walk the path along the river twice a day.

It's a pleasant walk on a summer afternoon. I put on a blue gingham dress I made for myself. It has a full gathered skirt and a narrow pink velvet ribbon sash, and it's the first time I've worn it. Life feels great—wonderful summer evening, a new dress, people I enjoy to socialize with, and a Huxley in town. Francis, a social anthropologist with endless originality, has added a lot of stimulation to our life here.

I'm first to arrive at the cottage and, when I remark on that, Francis says, "There may not be anyone else showing up." That's odd. People usually gather wherever Francis is these days. He asks me if I'd like a cup of tea, and when I accept he suddenly seems to change his mind and says, "Or would you rather have LSD?"

I think he's joking, but he seems rather serious about it. I remind him that I'm forbidden to take LSD, on orders from headquarters, since Dr. Osmond is worried that I might get into a space I couldn't get out of. I've had a breakdown and Dr. Osmond is insistent that anyone who may show the least sign of instability not be given LSD.

I say, "You know I'm curious to see how it compares to the real thing."

"You mean your own experiences. There's no such thing as 'the real thing,'" says Francis. I've learned a lot about mental fencing with a Huxley, so I don't try to argue the point. Should I press Francis to tell me whether or not he has permission to give me the drug? Oh, what the heck!

Francis is an insider in the research. He's not only taken it several times and written about it, he's been sitter with quite a few subjects. Dr. Osmond would trust him to make a decision like this.

I may know more about what's going on than most of the staff. Not only am I friendly with Francis Huxley, but I have a pal working in research. She tells me they've given LSD to a few of the staff members they weren't too confident about. There are people who may show a few abnormal symptoms but who, unlike me, haven't faced them yet. Nobody wants to tell a person bluntly, the way Dr. Osmond told me, that they might get lost in inner space, so they give them a minute dose. "What you do," my friend explained, "is dip your finger in LSD and wipe it on the inside of the glass."

Francis shoos me into the living room, so I don't see what he's doing about dosage. I suspect he's giving me the wiped glass. But I know I'm in good hands. If Francis thinks I can handle LSD, then it will be okay. I relax on the chesterfield, facing the picture window, drink the little medicine glass of water when he hands it to me, and settle down to talk and listen to music. Francis takes the big chair in the corner to my left. There is a standing lamp behind his chair.

I always find the Osmond living room delightful. They keep a set of bright brass angel chimes on top of the bookcase, year round, and the furnishings all express comfort and hominess. There is no pretension, just a wonderful sense of personalized uniqueness.

I've heard the onset of the drug is sudden, but I couldn't have imagined how sudden. One instant I am talking normally to Francis, and the next instant the lamp behind him is producing approximately the same amount of light as the sun. I wince and close my eyes, and Francis casually reaches up and turns off the lamp. That's the job of the sitter—to be there for the subject every instant, never letting your concentration stray, picking up on cues and making the journey as smooth as possible. And Francis is a pro. But turning off the standing lamp doesn't begin to end the sharply enhanced perception I'm experiencing. Now I am drowning in the music. It has become unbearably loud and I'm lost in it. I want to swim in it, but I can't. It frustrates me. I don't know if I'm giving any signs, but Francis asks quietly, "Music bothering you?" He gets up and turns it down.

I become mesmerized by the angel chimes. Francis walks over and sets them spinning. They twinkle and tinkle, but they are metal. They reflect light. They seem to deflect me. My attention turns instead to the red rug. I've always loved that rug. I know of no one else who has a red rug in the living room. I don't mean a patterned rug and I don't mean a dark, wine-toned rug. The Osmond rug is a rich crimson red, exciting enough in any circumstances. Under LSD it is beyond description. I just sink into the rug, explore the recesses in the nap, feel it comforting me, hurting me, making my visual sense real. As I sit staring at the rug, the red is ingesting me, the music is swallowing me, and I am overcome by depression.

I've always seen myself as a helper, and I've always had satisfaction from that. But suddenly I feel resentful. I feel as if every request for advice or assistance has piled up on top of me, like an actual load. My talents have been useful, but where is the appreciation? Feelings of worthlessness leave me beyond forlorn. I lay my head against the back of the chesterfield. I suppose I want to cry, but I can't identify any feeling. I am wiped. The heaviness is so bad I can no longer hold myself up. I slip from my seat and crouch on the floor with my head on the couch, and I am nothing but suffering. No me. Just something negative and overwhelming.

Francis' voice is saying, "Get up, Kay." It is said gently, but it is a command. He is not going to let me wallow in self-contempt. I get up, but I feel mortified because, in slipping off the couch, my knee has caught the skirt of my new gingham dress and ripped about seven inches from the waistline seam. Soon after that, Francis gives me niacin to swallow. He doesn't want me to spiral into despair. As I climb slowly back to some kind of reality, the ripped dress brings a feeling of shame. Childish as it is, it makes me feel normal. My agitation probably shows, because Francis says, "Take peace, Kay." I must be extremely sensitive to suggestion, because I am able to find that peace.

༄

That is all I remember of my LSD experience. It was 1958, a long time ago. I took the drug around 6:45, and sometime around midnight I heard Francis asking if I'd like a cup of tea now. I said I would. I felt dazed, disoriented, and had little memory; yet when Francis remarked, "You have it now," I knew exactly what he meant. I could feel myself settling at some new level of understanding of self and other. We talked about what had happened and when I told Francis about my little bout of paranoia, of feeling so *used* by people, he answered without hesitation, "You may as well face it. You're one of the strong ones."

No wonder people reported achieving insight when under LSD. I got a totally new impression of myself in that instant, and it was to strengthen me many times through the years. I, who had considered myself a weakling, was one of the strong ones. It was a revelation.

Sometime about two a.m., Francis walked me home along the river road. Noticing that I was stepping gingerly, he asked, "Can you tell where the road is?" I answered,

"Yes, I know where the road is—I'm not sure where my feet are."

At my door, Francis ordered me to go straight to bed, and he emphasized, "Don't you leave this house tonight under any circumstances." I was back inside my own head sufficiently to hear what he said and I obeyed him, but I didn't take any of it in realistically. I was myself the next day. Francis phoned in the morning to check on that.

Research into the effects of LSD had been going on in Saskatchewan for five years by then. Dr. Humphry Osmond became superintendent of the hospital at Weyburn in 1953 and he was an eager partner for Dr. Abram Hoffer, head of psychiatric research for the province. Extremely innovative, Osmond provided a contrast to Hoffer's exacting scientific approach, but they complemented each other. Dr. Osmond had a theory that schizophrenia was caused by some biochemical imbalance in the body when adrenaline was breaking down. He was interested in mescaline, a derivative of the peyote cactus, and he and Dr. Hoffer attended a ceremony with an Aboriginal group so Dr. Osmond could take the drug. He was convinced the feelings of withdrawal and hallucinations he experienced were very similar to what was described by patients with schizophrenia. The doctors then found a pure source of LSD that they felt was suitable for experimentation. Because the Aboriginal people had taken it in a group setting, they wanted to use it in groups, but first they took it themselves, to get an idea of possible effects and how it might be controlled.

LSD could be a very unpleasant experience, unpredictable in the extreme and sometimes causing panic. It was never safe to leave a subject alone when they were under the drug. It was less stressful if the atmosphere was quiet and pleasant, so music and flowers were introduced. The sitter, who had not taken the drug, tried to guide the episode by asking questions, but nothing could really be done to determine the direction a "trip" would take. They found that a high dose of niacin would terminate the experience if it proved to be leading into dark places.

Those who took LSD in a group were usually senior staff like doctors, interns, psychologists, social workers, creative therapists, or senior nurses who had taken training in counselling. They were dedicated professionals, people who were willing to enter the frightening world inhabited by their patients if it would make them more effective in trying to help. Despite the fact that subjects were withdrawn while under the drug, they found it enhanced a feeling of empathy in those who went through the experience together. Better yet, the feeling lasted after the effects wore off. This was a double plus for people working in psychiatry, because it increased awareness of others while at the same time providing a new understanding of what it felt like to endure the distorted perceptions experienced by so many of the mentally ill.

Student nurses were not encouraged to take LSD, but a small handful of the very curious persuaded the authorities to let them try. I entered training in 1956, and my first encounter with LSD was witnessing, at a distance, someone under the effects. The girl was moving very slowly, taking ages to gaze at things. After a while she made a purposeful movement, walking straight into the river. The others did nothing to startle her, but they did watch carefully. The Souris River was gorgeous that day and I was trying to imagine how much more spectacular it must look to her, to make her want to wade in and blend with it like that. She watched the ripples spread with each step, and then she sat, suddenly, plunk, in the water. She picked up a leafy twig and began to splash the water with it slowly, watching the droplets fall.

The others hadn't encouraged or discouraged her, but now Francis spoke with a little more force, suggesting quietly she might get out of the river and they could take her where she could find dry clothes. When they were gone, I hurried over to where they had been standing, to see what added magic was on the water from that angle. To my horror, there was no silver sheen. It was an ugly, dirty, dark brown Souris, littered with dead things and silt. As I was watching, a water snake circled and raised its head exactly where the girl had been sitting. LSD creates illusions, but what an illusion that must have been!

The incident left me with a big question. I can imagine a patient looking at the beauty I saw and seeing instead a slough of muddy water and a snake. Maybe some patients could look at the dirty river and see beautiful scenery, but my guess is it wouldn't happen often. As far as I can see, lovely visions are not the most common stuff of hallucinations. Horrors are. So is LSD really allowing sane people to get a view of what the mentally ill experience? Distorted perception, yes, but without delusional context and without the twenty-four-hour-a-day process going on month after month, year after year. It didn't begin to compare with the years and years of distortion endured by so many of the mentally ill in those days.

Also, when I was ill, I had very little in the way of visual distortion. What I had was far too many hours of auditory hallucinations. It was also my observation while doing psychiatric nursing that auditory hallucinations far outweighed visual in most instances. I never heard an LSD subject report hearing voices. So, aside from the emotional "down," feeling of panic, and the fact that it distorted perception, I didn't feel that LSD really provided the model of psychosis researchers felt it did.

Whether LSD really increased empathy, no one could ever prove, but when I worked in psychiatry at University Hospital in Saskatoon I won a reputation as a good LSD sitter. A sitter had to be able to concentrate for at least eight straight hours. You couldn't let your mind wander from the subject, even for a moment, and this didn't mean simply watching behaviour. You had to intuit what the subject was feeling and experiencing from moment to moment. It was an intensely draining experience, but a very satisfying one. If my own little "trip" had something to do with it, then I know what Francis meant when he said, "You have it now."

By that time they had discovered that LSD was most effective in treating alcoholism, but its days of medical use were numbered. When Dr. Osmond went to California to give LSD to Aldous Huxley, and Huxley wrote his books about the drug, they made the mistake of talking to Timothy Leary about their hopes and plans. Unfortunately, Leary put a different spin on the story and LSD became part of the "hippie" age. By the mid-sixties, so much impure LSD was being given to unscreened subjects in dangerous circumstances that there was a hue and cry from the public. The drug could no longer be acquired, even by responsible doctors using it in controlled settings, and Saskatchewan had to discontinue its use.

Admittedly, the bit I took is hardly worthy to be called an experiment, but it is one experience I will never forget: I took LSD from a Huxley, the nephew of the very man who wrote *The Doors of Perception*. I have never been a stranger to serendipity.

LSD

The year was 1963. I'd been "sitting" an LSD since 8 o'clock that morning. My patient was actually a nurse, one of my colleagues, and she had been admitted for just one day in order to have an LSD experience. We were working on the psychiatric unit of University Hospital in Saskatoon. When it came to progressive psychiatry in the fifties, Saskatchewan was out in front. My subject, like most of our professional staff who had taken LSD, wanted to find out how her patients felt, what it was like to have the senses distorted, to lose control of your own mind. She had listed a secondary purpose for taking the drug: she wanted to see if it would enhance her self-awareness. Like most of us, she had some insecurities and anxieties, and she had high hopes for what might happen under LSD.

It had been a quiet experience. She spent hours gazing at plants and a mark on the wall. Now and then she answered questions with a nod. She refused her dinner tray. We used the handbook by Duncan Blewett and N. Chwelos as a general guide when sitting an LSD experience, and this experience was following the predictable pattern, but in a very quiet and uninvolved sort of way. At about four o'clock, as expected, the effects began to lift and my patient smiled and seemed ready to talk. I asked her how it went and she relayed a few of her experiences, but she wasn't quite herself. She acted confused and slightly suspicious. When her husband arrived to have her discharged and take her home for the night, she suddenly turned to me and blurted, "Can you come home with me?"

It was the first time I'd had a request like that, but when you agree to sit an LSD you agree to a commitment. As long as the subject needs you, you are there. So the three of us went "home" together, and I was to be there all evening and far into the night. Her husband made supper, and then we sat in the living room carrying on a pleasant conversation. She told us she wasn't ready to say much about the experience yet. After a while she seemed so normal I suggested I should leave and let them get to bed, but she shook her head vigorously and insisted I not leave. It was about two a.m. when she put a tentative hand on her husband's knee and felt the cloth of his pants the way a child might explore a strange toy. After a moment she smiled and said, "You can go home now if you want to, Parley. He still doesn't look like himself, but he's starting to feel like himself."

∾

Being a psychiatric nurse in Saskatchewan at that time was exciting, and I was thrilled when colleagues began to refer to me as an LSD "specialist." I did see quite a lot of it. I was one of the sitters for a problem patient who took mescaline experimentally at Weyburn, and that introduced me to the unpredictability of the drug. I never knew, when she was brought home to the ward to my care after her session, whether she would be childish and silly, withdrawn and nervous, weeping hysterically or broken-heartedly. I sat with one young man who asked to have me as his sitter three times. The first two were positive, but his third was a "bad trip." He told me later he felt as if there was a box up in the corner of his room and he was trapped inside it and I wasn't letting him out. Perhaps I'd asked too many questions. We always discussed such matters with the subject ahead of time, and any questions I asked would have been his own suggestions, but a nurse sitting an LSD learned to keep quiet by the hour. In any event, it ruined my relationship with the young man for more than two weeks. He seemed to be paranoid about me and wouldn't speak. Later he confessed it was all because I asked one of the orderlies to accompany him to the washroom. Spaced out as he was, he still figured he could have been trusted to go to the washroom alone, and it turned him away from me on the instant. That's how vulnerable a subject under LSD could be. A raised eyebrow could be enough to change the mood from sunny to gloomy. A sitter required vast stores of empathy. Like anyone involved with medical research using LSD, I was no admirer of Timothy Leary, but he did say something about LSD sitters that was right on. In *Politics of Ecstasy* Leary wrote, "A new profession of psychedelic guides will inevitably develop to supervise these experiences. The training for this new profession will aim at producing the patience of a first-grade teacher, the humility and wisdom of a Hindu guru, the loving dedication of a minister-priest, the sensitivity of a poet, and the imagination of a science fiction writer." He was right. We would sit for eight hours a day, concentrating all our energy on someone who was uncommunicative. There was usually a gap of three or four hours when they didn't talk at all. It was like being in a room with someone engrossed in their own book, but if you let your attention leave their mind for an instant the book will change for them and possibly lead them into despair. The sitter's interest and attention are the subject's lifeline. They have lost their ego. You are it. They have lost their sense of direction. You are their guide. They are drifting in space. You are there to bring them back to earth. It is a great growing experience for a sitter, if exhausting. It is the most intuitive and empathic relationship I have ever known. I found that the very concentration freed me of self and produced a state of relaxation akin to the state I often achieve when painting. It's a state in which the world fails to intrude.

LSD could leave residual effects, and depression was one of them. Our doctors were meticulously careful about who took the drug. It was known to be nonaddictive and had no side effects except for occasional nausea, but it did produce lasting emotional wallops. We never gave it to anyone with schizophrenia. What would be the point of making a sick person sicker? Subjects were checked for liver damage and were well informed. They knew the chances they were taking and were willing and even eager to take them. Most of the subjects were alcoholics because it was soon evident that many alcoholics really benefitted from an LSD experience. Occasionally we would admit someone from as far away as New York who had come to Saskatoon to take LSD from Dr. Hoffer. Motivation was important. A subject was expected to have a clearly stated purpose for the experience, and that experience would be tightly controlled. Subjects spent the entire day in a closed room, most of the time with only their sitter, but the doctor would come in occasionally. If someone was scheduled to relieve the sitter for lunch or coffee break, that would be arranged the day before so the subject would not be exposed to any surprises. Sometimes I was so involved in a session that I stayed in the room for lunch.

There was a general belief that the best sitters were people who had had the experience of taking LSD, and my fellow nurses asked where I got my empathy for subjects, because I never told them I'd taken it. Dr. Osmond had forbidden me to try LSD, but Francis Huxley got permission to give me the enormous dose of 5 mcg one evening. (We usually gave 100 to 400 mcg, so my indoctrination was slight.) That may be where I learned how to sit an LSD, but any aptitude I showed for the role could also have come from other sources. Most of my colleagues concluded that my experience of a real mental breakdown had led to considerable empathy for people undergoing the treatment. I also had some training in drama and had spent quite a bit of time involved in theatre work. I don't think the actor's art hurt me at all when it came to developing empathy for someone under LSD.

Whatever the reason, I became in demand. My article on the nurse's role, "Supporting the Patient on LSD Day," appeared in *The American Journal of Nursing,* February, 1964, and is the next chapter in this book. I don't know of any other articles on the nurse's role published at the time. When a psychiatrist and two nurses asked me to be their sitter when they took LSD as a group, I felt I had hit the pinnacle of my career, but vacation time intervened and I missed the opportunity. I have always regretted that I never saw LSD used in a group situation.

Sometimes I wonder if I would have burned out as an LSD nurse. It was such an exhausting thing. I always felt as if I'd just been on stage in a play that ran eight hours—totally drained when it was over.

At the time we were using LSD there was little fear of the drug. Whereas drugs such as heroin and opium seemed to destroy conscience, LSD seemed to improve it. It enhanced sensory perception, it could increase self-awareness and expand mental horizons. But it was very unpredictable, and our doctors used it very cautiously. In Saskatchewan, I never heard of anyone being given one of the overpowering doses of 2,000 mcg and I never knew of a patient being given the drug without knowledge and consent. Much of the time our doctors and other psychiatric staff were using themselves, not our patients, as guinea pigs. The worst experience we ever witnessed occurred in a girl who became so panicky she curled up in the corner of her bed and refused to let anyone near her. She also tried to throw herself from a fourth floor window. She was given a hurried dose of niacin IV, which reduced the effects of LSD rapidly. I never saw violence. I did hear of one male patient who made a pass at his nurse.

That night in 1963 when I went home with my fellow nurse to lend her security until she recognized her husband again, we had no inkling that within three years LSD would be the bad guy of the North American continent. Erika Dyck gives a thorough history of the spread of panic and its aftermath in her book *Psychedelic Psychiatry: LSD from Clinic to Campus* (Johns Hopkins University Press, 2008). It was certainly one of the most dramatic stories of our century. Creative artists of several stripes latched on to LSD as something to enhance experience, the popularity of the drug spread to the daring young people on the university campuses, and the drug literally became epidemic. Worst of all, cheap substitutes and even homemade varieties began to be used and were far more dangerous than the pure LSD used in medical experiments. The carefully planned and supervised sessions with trained experts weren't available to the thousands of young people now spreading "acid" lavishly across the map. Not surprisingly, the media saw a very dramatic story and rode to battle against LSD, concentrating on the bizarre and ignoring the cautious, careful scientific work that had been going on in various psychiatric centres. The result was that doctors lost control of LSD and it ended up under the jurisdiction of the law; and the law, as Charles Dickens knew so well, is an ass, especially when, as seems to have been the case here, legislation is based not on scientific investigation but on what appears in magazines and on TV.

Probably most of the fear of LSD was really fear of psychosis. Many people don't want to be insane even temporarily. That is a fear I don't really share. I think a temporary psychosis would do a lot of people a lot of good. They might come out of it with more insight into the real madness around us—the madness of polluting the environment, poisoning food supplies, destroying ozone layers, and stockpiling weapons to blow the world up forty-eight times while children weep for food and medical care. That is psychosis, not the experience of someone on a "trip."

Despite my refusal to panic over the thought of LSD, I do recognize the dangers. I understand the red-light phenomenon—the LSD taker who, looking at a red light, sees the beauty of it filling his world and drives up and into it as into paradise, never realizing it is a stop sign. It could happen. It could happen that someone on LSD might walk off a high building, unaware of danger. Police had a right to be concerned. As I mentioned earlier, I once witnessed an LSD experience when a young woman who had taken the drug walked into the Souris River and sat down in the water, enthralled by the ripples and oblivious to possible danger. Of course her sitter was there, watching every move. The people who used LSD in those days of experimentation in Saskatchewan were not fools. They were very very cautious and very very organized.

I've seen quite a lot of LSD. I loved working with it. There was a time when I thought it might be a giant step to a higher consciousness, and it's rather a pity it didn't prove to be the Pegasus we once thought it was. But I still feel grateful that psychiatry discovered LSD, if only for a decade, because it led to so much more understanding of the mentally ill. I spent the years 1949 to 1956 in the suspect land of those who are stigmatized because they have suffered a nervous breakdown. I dared not talk about hallucinatory experiences to anyone because it scared them half to death. Professionals were the worst because they'd conclude I needed treatment.

Then psychiatrists began to experiment with LSD, and for the very first time I found I could relax with them and talk about my adventures in inner space without making them panic. When I worked with fellow nurses who had taken LSD, I found them easier to relate to and easier to work with in our approach to patients. LSD was such an indirect boon to me that I can't help feeling thankful to the drug to this day. Once upon a time a few daring humans found a way to expand the mind. Were they crazy? Who knows? The real question is, "Was it wise to shut it down?"

SUPPORTING THE
PATIENT ON LSD DAY

My experience with LSD, both as one who had taken the drug and as a nurse-sitter, led me to write an article that appeared in the American Journal of Nursing *in 1964. An edited version of the article is reprinted here.*

എ

No role is so welcomed on our psychiatric unit as that of "sitting" with a patient during LSD therapy. This indicates that the treatment has value because nurses tend to like whatever gives them satisfaction. The psychiatric nurse appreciates a situation that provides an opportunity for her to form constructive personal relationships with her patients. She likes to be involved in treatments that give her patients the most benefit with the least mental or physical discomfort, and she enjoys seeing results from her work. Anyone who has watched LSD properly used knows LSD is rewarding in all these areas.

It is not the purpose of this article to advance arguments for or against this controversial drug. Ours was a research hospital where LSD was cautiously prescribed and studied during its therapeutic use. Although it was used chiefly for alcoholic patients, there are others who derived benefit from it. Many alcoholic patients requested LSD because they had heard or read of it, or had had previous treatments. They were tested physically and psychologically, and oriented to the treatment by a psychiatrist. It was never administered without the patient's active consent.

Where possible the patient should be allowed his choice of nurse to sit with him during the experience. A patient under LSD is often very sensitive and can easily suffer a sense of rejection or become suspicious. He requires expert guidance from an understanding companion. Also, he is apt to uncover deep emotional problems that can be endured better in the company of someone with whom he feels at ease. A patient under LSD should never be left alone for an instant because a world of fear, anxiety, and unreality could beset the solitary individual.

The nurse chosen by the patient should try to spend considerable time with her patient the day before treatment, encouraging him to discuss the problems he hopes to solve and asking questions about his fears or doubts. The patient for whom LSD is prescribed is almost invariably rational and able to express himself clearly. Even so, it is difficult to explain the drug's action to the uninitiated. For one thing, LSD's precise effect cannot be anticipated because it differs with each individual.

However, we can predict that LSD may expand the patient's concept of space and time, enable him to scan his life and perhaps to concentrate on forgotten events and see them in new perspective. LSD may intensify past experiences and bring new meaning to relationships with other people. We can warn the patient that he may become depressed, suspicious, and even suicidal, that he may behold vast beauty and color, or ugliness, horror, and despair. We can suggest that he may reach the root of the problem that has caused his drinking—that he may even be able to plan his future with fresh insight and a new sense of proportion. Often, because he already knows where his problems lie, he asks the nurse to focus his attention on this area. Frequently he expects LSD will allow him to step *outside* himself and view himself objectively. Sometimes this happens.

In the preliminary period and during treatment, most patients require considerable reassurance. Some are afraid of the unknown; some are afraid of themselves.

One patient was very tense because he thought he would become violently hostile under LSD, as he did when drunk. On the contrary, after LSD took effect, he lay on his bed weeping because his father hadn't shown him affection as a child. The nurse should assure her patient that she will be with him constantly, that his physician will be with him as much as is necessary, and that the drug, which is given in the morning, will wear off at about 4:00.

Because LSD offers a unique opportunity to the adventurous, some people are more excited than apprehensive. Since John Glenn orbited the universe, it has been easier to orient a patient to LSD treatment. The two concepts are similar in that an astronaut conquers outer space, while recipients of the "mind-manifester" try the limits of inner space.

"You are off on a trip," I have told them, "with no baggage, no destination, and no compass. That's why I'm here. I can't go with you, but I can be your anchor. Wherever you go, you'll always be able to see me. I'll be the nurse who sits beside your bed, taking notes and playing your records. You'll never lose touch with me. Seeing me, you'll know you are really in hospital and that you'll be back to earth about four o'clock. I will send you signals, too, to encourage your explorations. I will remind you of places you longed to revisit and events you hoped to scan."

Other preparations include choosing music and borrowing the records requested by the patient. The nurse who will make possible our coffee and dinner breaks is introduced. If she is not available the previous day, she meets the patient in the morning before he takes the drug, because he should know, so far as possible, what to expect: after LSD takes effect, strangers or unforeseen events can be very disconcerting. Showing keen interest in "tomorrow," we say good night with promises of enthusiastic cooperation. This is remarkably easy. The nurse's chief difficulty lies in curbing her own excitement enough to get a good night's sleep.

The nurse-patient relationship during LSD treatment is, I suspect, like that between partners on a mountain-climbing team—warm, cooperative, intimate, and yet objective. This highly motivated partnership is welcome because it does not resemble the sticky, emotional "involvements" that psychiatric nurses must shun. This is a team going someplace!

"Concentrate on your patient," I tell student nurses who are preparing to "sit." "Don't let your mind leave him for a second, all day long. Above all, relax. You are his security. Tension in you will create tensions in him that will set up blockades against the drug and cause him hideous experiences that won't be useful to him. *Concentrate* and *relax.*"

"But," one student complained, "I don't understand. If I'm to concentrate so hard, how can I possibly relax? The two contradict each other!"

I was glad she had presented this puzzle. To explain the treatment to someone who had never experienced it, I fell back on the theatre.

Luckily, this student had acted.

"It's that kind of relaxation," I explained. "You know your role, you're all concentration. In reality you are tense, keyed up, every nerve on edge. But the moment you step on stage, you relax by forgetting yourself entirely and concentrating your whole attention outside yourself. Throughout the LSD treatment, all that nervous energy must flow to your patient. At four o'clock you'll be completely exhausted but wildly exultant—then you'll realize that you were relaxed. There are few satisfactions to equal completing a whole day with an LSD patient. It's like coming off stage after a good performance!"

On the morning of the treatment, the nurse makes sure that her patient is washed, dressed, shaved, and in a quiet single room. His bed is made and the stands left tidy. If possible we add a bouquet of flowers because the LSD patient should be surrounded by calm and beauty. He has only coffee for breakfast as nausea and vomiting sometimes occur. They are the only side effects of LSD that we have encountered. The nurse suffers none of the apprehensions of nurses caring for patients who receive electric shock or insulin therapy. There will be no change in vital signs, no seizures, no alarming developments whatsoever. Supplies include an emesis basin, box of tissues, record player, and the patient's choice of records, paper, pencils, and a clipboard. The patient understands that his nurse will note any important things he says or any emotional changes he shows that may be of use to him and his doctor.

These preparations are completed by 8:30 or 9:00 a.m. Then the doctor administers the LSD, a liquid, orally, in water. Dosage ranges from 100 to 400 micrograms. After the patient drinks the medicine, doctor and nurse wish him luck. Usually the physician leaves the room until the drug has begun to take effect in about thirty to forty-five minutes. Patient and nurse are off on their adventure. Sometimes they start the music. Sometimes they just chat.

Presently the patient may forget to answer a question or say that he feels "different" or "a bit apprehensive." Time and remark are noted. Whether he lies quietly, sits up, talks ceaselessly, laughs, weeps, tries to disguise his feelings, or is unbelievably honest—whatever happens, the nurse records his moods. She answers when he speaks, and talks to him if she feels his silence is not constructive. The day goes very rapidly for her, though it can seem endless to the patient, who may have temporarily lost his sense of time. One must rely heavily on intuition, for like someone with schizophrenia, a patient under LSD can be extremely reticent or may communicate in a very distorted fashion.

Yet the nurse develops a feeling whether this LSD experience is a "good one" or not. When the doctor participates extensively it is easier to judge, because then the nurse can observe and see better the direction the experience is taking. When she emerges for lunch, she invariably is asked, "How is it? Is it a good one?" This is the other ward staff's only chance to hear news of the patient because no one enters the room unless so arranged by patient and doctor.

Recently at noon a student came out of an LSD treatment room so tired her knees were buckling. "I've been concentrating so *hard!* I don't know how I'll live 'til the end of the day!"

At four o'clock she was both weary and exultant. It had been a "good" LSD. Next day her patient said the nurse was "an angel to me all day."

This appreciation is probably one reason we like to "sit." We forget self, we drain our mental reserves, we empathize until we wonder who is having the LSD, the patient or the nurse; we go home dizzy with fatigue but happy, and the next day the patient tells his friends that he couldn't have gone through it without his nurse.

LSD is a direct route to establishing relationships with patients. One comes closer to depths of human understanding and emotion than one has ever been. Once I watched an LSD patient's basic personality problem iron itself out before my eyes, with a magic unknown except in fairy tales. Because of this unique relationship between patient and nurse, we often spend part of the evening discussing the day's events with the patient after LSD has worn off. A nurse who was not present could not be as helpful. I have worked fourteen hours at a stretch with an LSD treatment, and felt the time well spent.

It is not surprising that unimaginative thinkers have reservations about LSD. Not only does it lead man's mind into realms of time and space where people have always hesitated to go, but LSD forms ties that must seem "superstitious" to those who have not seen the drug in use. These ties are fairly well understood by our nursing personnel. We accept the idea that we can "feel" our way through the treatment and that we can "feel" the effect LSD is having on the patient. We agree that a patient must choose his nurse and that a nurse must be free to sit, or refuse to sit, with him. This whole area, like drama, requires intuitive creativity. After several exposures to it, one's sensitivity becomes almost uncanny. Practically any nurse on the ward can anticipate which nurse will want to sit with the next LSD and find that she has guessed correctly. Not uncommonly, a nurse explains that, because she just sat with an LSD, she must rebuild her energy before she sits with another. Or she may say, "I'm saving myself for Monday. If I sat now, I'd be depleted."

Superstition or another step toward enlightenment? We don't know. We do know that we found our part in LSD therapy rewarding, and we worked gladly with this adjunct to psychiatric therapy. Our graduate nurses described their position in LSD therapy as that of "a companion, an anchor, a guide, someone to give the patient reassurance, to focus his attention on his problems, to keep him in touch with reality, to work through his emotional traumas with him and give him understanding."

No nurse implied that her role was merely to observe the patient and take notes. And no one suggested calling the nurse "a believer." Those of us who worked closely with this controversial drug never sat down and asked ourselves whether we believe in it or not. If it is going to be used at all, it should be skilfully and with the greatest possible benefit to the patient.

THE WEYBURN THAT WAS

When Dr. Abram Hoffer first saw the mental hospital at Weyburn, he called it the worst mental hospital he'd ever seen. That was in about 1950. When I spent the winter of 1948–49 there as a patient, I found it a very good hospital. I had good psychiatrists and the chance to participate in lots of recreational activities. I spent five months editing the in-house paper, *The Torch* and even had hypnotherapy and was given a psychodrama, sophisticated treatments in psychiatry in those days. Group therapy was started while I was there, and the group had both male and female patients from the admission wards. We had discussions and plenty of social and recreational life. Movies, dances, and concerts were a regular feature in the assembly hall, and the members of the psychotherapy group actually had a lot of fun.

So what's going on here? I've just described an excellent treatment hospital in the very institution Dr. Hoffer described as the worst he ever saw. Well, that good hospital existed, but it existed on only two wards in that whole enormous building: the male and female admission units.

The hospital at Weyburn was established circa 1921 and was based on the pattern that had been refined in the Victorian age. The Victorians were a hard-headed and practical lot, and they were also elitist. You didn't waste education on the boy with limited intelligence because you needed the best minds in leadership positions. Similarly, you didn't waste time trying to cure a "hopeless" mental patient. You picked those who showed potential for recovery and concentrated on them. That was still the way it was in the late 1940s—and, for me, it worked. They kept promising patients on the admission wards for six months. If you weren't well by then you were likely to be transferred. They kept me on admission for nine months and that made all the difference, because when I left hospital I never had to go back and I've led a pretty productive life. I like to say, "They did a pretty good job on me!"

There was little therapy on any other ward. If you were well enough to be one of the workers who kept the place going—if you could work on farm or yard gang, in laundry or sewing room, help in kitchen or dining rooms, or even earn your keep by scrubbing washrooms and floors— then you might live on a workers' ward and they tried to treat workers well. They got better food, their wards were quiet compared to units where the more violent patients were housed, and they got to participate in all of the sports and entertainment. Parole patients were free to spend lots of time out of doors, and several of them grew gardens. That was not only marvellous therapy, it provided them with fresh vegetables to give them a healthier diet. But if you count activity shared with professional personnel who were paying attention to you as an individual, there wasn't any real therapy on workers' wards. There were only enough psychiatrists and psychologists to see patients on the admission wards. The other patients were watched, fed, and kept clean and, if they became physically ill, they were treated. The hospital had two adequate "sick wards" and even their own surgery. But life on most of the units was stagnant.

What had caused Weyburn to fall into a situation where its reputation was so poor? When it was built, it was considered one of the best mental hospitals in the country. It was beautifully designed, spacious, well lighted, and it had wonderful grounds with the Souris River winding through them. There were lovely lawns and flowerbeds.

It had a ball diamond, skating and curling rinks, and room for all kinds of activity. Still, the problems began in those days. In the twenties, a mental hospital existed to hide the mentally ill from society, an enforced segregation that only served to reinforce fear of the illness and increase the stigma. The goal was to keep patients quiet and peaceful, exert control, and, above all, permit no behaviour that might offend the middle-class definition of "normal." Any nurse in authority was an RN and adhered to general hospital ideals: cleanliness, order, routine, and every patient in his designated place. The rest of the staff were inadequately trained and understood psychiatry as being a matter of control. It was chiefly about making people behave. Keeping them clean, fed, and in reasonable health was important, and that was seen to with a kind of military discipline. Even though training for ward staff gradually became longer and a bit more enlightened, antiquated attitudes persisted right up to the mid-forties. Even then, there were still supervisors on many of the wards whose attitudes had atrophied.

In the beginning, in the 1920s, clean and sparse furnishings on a shiny floor were the ideal environment. Chairs were lined up in straight rows and patients were supposed to sit where they were put. Orderliness was the name of the game. When the hospital was being revitalized in the early fifties, a researcher took some photos of the wards and some of the units were still following that pattern. Chairs were not only lined up in rows, but back to back, and one photo showed two silent regressed women with schizophrenia seated side by side (no communication), and back to back with similar patients in chairs behind them. After all, putting the chairs in a circle and encouraging conversation would have created a stir. The ward could have been noisy. It would have made it more difficult for the nurses to control behaviour. Lawdy lawdy. That was the old Weyburn. That was the hospital that existed in 1948–49 when I was a patient there. Thank goodness the admission wards were progressive, and thank goodness I was never moved off admission.

When I was in training, from 1956 to 1959, noise and stir were givens. Encouraging normal human interaction is what it was all about. We had an early tranquilizer, Largactil, and it was the first "magic bullet." Without it, many of the patients would still have been unapproachable most of the time. Science was beginning to catch up, and by then the Weyburn hospital was in a position to take advantage of that.

Did I see anything good about the *old* hospital—aside from the enlightened treatments I received? As a matter of fact, I did. The medieval idea of isolating the mentally ill had evolved in the nineteenth century into an ideal in which society should provide a decent place where all of those misfits could live together. There would be "sane" staff to keep things running smoothly, and health care and entertainment. What resulted was a segregated community, but *it was a community*. People made friends there. Patients who were well enough showed initiative whenever they could. The more relaxed members of the staff were on quite friendly terms with some of the patients. Best of all, the work patients did was seen as a contribution. As I said about my work on the *Torch* in an article in *Transition*, Spring 2006, "By asking me to play a creative and responsible role in a project which involved supposedly normal individuals working with patients, I was given the opportunity to see myself as a contributing member of society once more. I find it discouraging that the medical model has led psychiatry to a position of 'You are sick. I can help you,' when what is needed is a sense of 'You can help me. You can contribute to the community.'"

But *why* had the Weyburn hospital, which started out with so much promise, deteriorated into the subhuman conditions to be found there in the thirties and forties? The major problem was that Saskatchewan was harder hit by the dirty thirties than any other part of Canada. Not only was there little money to keep up staff or building, there were also far too many patients. Worry and poor diet caused so many mental breakdowns that by the end of that awful decade the building was clogged with patients.

It is also tragic that the hospital housed both those with intellectual disabilities and those with psychoses, which is not a good mixture. Slow learners need routine, whereas people with schizophrenia need variety in experience. Slow learners find it impossible to understand anything as complex and maddening as schizophrenia, and many suffering with psychoses have no patience with anyone who is slow. When the training school was built, most of the intellectually handicapped were taken out of the Weyburn mental hospital and staff were then free to concentrate on those with psychoses. (Quite a few of those with intellectual disabilities remained, because they were already trained and were some of the best workers in the place. They went on helping on the farm or yard gangs, trundling laundry and other necessary loads, serving meals and scrubbing floors. They were often better workers than those with psychoses, and were tolerated well.)

There was at least one other major problem that led to the bad reputation the hospital had during its second and third decades. That was lack of vision. Hope hardly existed. There was a superintendent who really held things back for years. He was a nice man. He knew the patients and made them feel at home. He was kindly and human—at least that is the persona he projected—but he could see no way of improving things. He simply adjusted to the status quo.

Those problems were all in existence in the winter of 1948–49, but there were signs of change. The training program for nurses had been expanded in 1947 from two years to three, and students were being given lots of new and positive ideas. I remember disliking several of the grads, because they were bossy and had so little feeling of empathy, but many of the student nurses were making the place liveable. They were proud to be training for the new profession of psychiatric nurse, but they were frustrated because so few of the supervisors would let them actually use the new ideas they were learning about in class. Neil McCallum, who later became a successful actor in England, was in second-year training when I was a patient and I knew him well. A sensitive man who loved to think outside of the box, Neil was one of the most frustrated. I remember the day he came to my *Torch* office to tell me they'd just had a lecture about change of method. He said, "What they don't realize is that what this place needs is not a change of method but a change of heart."

It was remarks like that from students like Neil that made my stay in Weyburn bearable. That and the psychiatrists, who were great. And of course the wonderful psychotherapy group and the psychologist who led it. Not to mention my "job" editing the *Torch*. If I think about it, I can certainly find a lot of very good things about The Mental at the end of the forties.

Another positive change happened in the forties—the boys came back from fighting World War II. In later years, one of the male staff remarked that there weren't many jobs for them when they came home, but they could get work at the mental hospital, so they did. Those fellows had learned to operate under tight discipline, do their duty, and keep their heads. A psychiatric ward was no doubt a snap after what they'd been through. Perhaps the male staff were okay before that (though I doubt it, from tales I have heard of violence and abuse), but the coming of the ex-service men certainly made a difference. The male side had a reputation for being more relaxed than the female wards. Men could handle emergencies with more ease. Maybe they just didn't get as worked up about things, but I know that when they began to book female nurses to the male wards, the female students often commented on how much more relaxed it was on the male side. The men were less fussy, less uptight, and they managed to sense when a patient could be allowed more initiative.

Still, nothing could really change under the old administration. The superintendent lacked long-term goals. Government was not keen on recognizing the need for spending on mental hospitals. Also, there was an entrenched bureaucratic structure. Promotion was based on seniority, so the nurse who had been on staff longest was in charge, regardless of his or her qualifications. Like the patients, nurses had to accept the fact that, when you work for a kind of police state, all you can do is stay out of trouble and keep your mouth shut.

But then the miracle happened. Tommy Douglas knew Weyburn and he was willing to ensure that his government gave mental patients a decent shot at life. Dr. McKerracher went to bat to light a fire under psychiatric services. Dr. Abram Hoffer took over the newly founded psychiatric research unit with qualifications and enthusiasm beyond anything Saskatchewan had ever experienced in the psychiatric field. And Dr. Humphry Osmond was appointed superintendent of the newly named Saskatchewan Hospital at Weyburn. That was the key that opened the locks. Here was a man of vision indeed, a brilliant man with a twenty-first century mind who was out to improve conditions for the mentally ill while simultaneously helping Dr. Hoffer find out what was wrong with them and what effective treatments could be discovered. Dr. Osmond came to Weyburn in 1951, became superintendent of the hospital in 1952, and in 1957, as stated earlier, the hospital won the American Psychiatric Association award as the North American mental hospital making the most progress. That was fast work. The hospital experienced what Neil McCallum had wished for in 1949: a change of heart.

The wards got a bright new look. There were more trained therapists. Suddenly every ward in the place was a treatment unit. Once violent patients on refractory wards were in groups. Patients with dementia were getting passive exercise and parties. The old workers' wards became continued treatment wards where, even though many continued to work as before, they were also involved in creative therapies and a variety of hands-on activities. They also received a bit of spending money as payment for their work. Best of all, doctors were now seeing some patients who had been moved off admissions. Since there still weren't enough psychiatrists to look after such a huge population, a number of graduate psychiatric nurses had taken clinical training and were doing therapy with longer-term patients.

A few of the old-time supervisors offered resistance and they couldn't be fired, but the new administration was smart. When they began the ward activities program, taking quantities of craft supplies and an occupational therapist right on to the wards, they began it on a ward where one of the hard-line supervisors wanted every patient seated in the same chair all day, out of the way and quiet. She quit. That, of course, was the whole idea.

However, if some patients were able to leave hospital and live in the community, half of the credit must go to society itself. The glorious sixties saw far stranger sights on our streets and in our parks than in our mental hospitals. Had the trend continued, we would have seen the day when the mental hospital would have been the only conformist society and the eccentrics would all have been on the outside. In the fifties, we had a patient in our hospital who dressed like a gypsy in a green and black dress with a scarlet kerchief on her head. She tied pink rags around her legs, carried a string bag full of a peculiar assortment of belongings, and pasted postage stamps on her face. In the sixties, there was a photograph of a group of hippies on the cover of a national magazine that made our patient look square.

The sixties were the greatest thing that could have happened to mental patients. It was much more than just this surface exhibition. There was interest in mind expansion and hallucinatory experiences, trends that anyone sincerely interested in the welfare of the mentally ill might have hailed with glee. It was a very real broadening of the base of tolerance. The children of the sixties were setting out to create a society that would make oddballs feel at home, and the mentally ill needed such a society. However, despite such changes, many patients weren't able to adjust to living outside the hospital. For example, I worked intensively with seven women on a high-level continued treatment unit. Their prospects were better than ninety percent of our hospital population. Yet only three were able, on discharge, to earn a living and take responsibility for their own lives, even part of the time.

In Dr. Osmond's day, patients who might be candidates for life in the community were chosen with care and given an extended period of re-training. They were informed of the changes that had taken place during the long years they had spent in hospital. They learned to use telephones again, go shopping on their own, and live on a ward with an open door. If it looked as if they could make the adjustment, they were tried on the boarding-out program. But as soon as psychiatry demonstrated some success in rehabilitating long-term patients, governments seem to have abdicated responsibility. A few years later, a new government was simply dumping patients onto communities and families who were often ill-equipped to deal with them. I actually heard of a government order to discharge eleven patients per week, regardless of their ability to function.

It was not quite as bad as it sounds. Support systems were in place to assist patients living in the community, but patients did not always see the need for them. Partially, it was a matter of the time factor. It takes a lot of time to get psychiatric patients oriented to a system, and time was no longer available. As a result, many people suffering with schizophrenia have fallen through the cracks and roam our streets, sometimes freezing to death on winter nights. It is like a nightmare from the Dark Ages.

Nowadays, when an ex-patient becomes violent or commits suicide, there is an instantaneous rationale: "He didn't take his medication." Drugs have become a means of bypassing the time-consuming and expensive therapies we used to use. They have reduced alternatives, and that is never wise. The proper use of drugs is to make it possible for therapists to work with a patient. Psychoactive drugs turned mental hospital hells into something no worse than purgatory. But they are a means of control. It is not difficult to envision a repressive regime in which mind-altering drugs are used to quiet all dissent, to shape the population into just what the system demands. Of course I can hardly be expected to greet drugs as the greatest thing that ever happened to psychiatry. I am the woman who threw Huxley's *Brave New World* across the room and hit the wall with it.

Despite my bias, I recognize that newer anti-psychotic medication has revolutionized psychiatry. Also, the need for family and community involvement has become better recognized. There was no Schizophrenia Society of Saskatchewan when I was first on the wards, but it began soon afterwards. The research that Dr. Abram Hoffer and Dr. Humphry Osmond were spearheading in Saskatchewan led to a treatment approach based on four principles: shelter, good food, respect, and what they termed the orthomolecular program. They discovered that patients with schizophrenia responded favourably to high doses of niacin, along with vitamin C and other essential nutrients.

How different many patients' lives might have been had they received that treatment when they first became ill. When I think of the millions of mentally ill humans whose potential was never realized and whose lives were filled with untold misery in so many societies over so many centuries, all I can say is, "What a waste."

ABOUT THE AUTHOR

During a varied life, Kay Parley has been an artist, school-teacher, and secretary. She graduated as a registered psychiatric nurse and holds the degrees of Bachelor of Arts with honours in sociology and Bachelor of Education from the University of Saskatchewan. She has devoted much time and study to writing and is a graduate of Lorne Greene's Academy of Radio Arts, Toronto (1948). She has published over forty stories and articles about the mentally ill and those who nurse them. Kay taught social sciences at Kelsey Institute in Saskatoon for eighteen years, retiring in 1987. She now writes steadily, with an emphasis on history and folklore. She has also written a community history, *They Cast a Long Shadow: The History of Moffat, Saskatchewan*.

THE REGINA COLLECTION

Named as a tribute to Saskatchewan's capital city and its rich history of boundary-defying innovation, The Regina Collection builds upon our motto of "a voice for many peoples," with these beautifully-packaged books by people caught up in social and political circumstances beyond their control.

Other books in *The Regina Collection:*

Time Will Say Nothing
by Ramin Jahanbegloo
(2014)

The Education of Augie Merasty
by Joseph Auguste Merasty,
with David Carpenter
(2015)

A NOTE ON THE TYPE

This body of this book is set in Adobe Garamond Pro. An Adobe Originals design, and Adobe's first historical revival, Adobe Garamond is a digital interpretation of the roman types of Claude Garamond (1480–1561) and the italic types of Garamond's assistant, Robert Granjon.

Designed by Robert Slimbach in 1989, Adobe Garamond has become a typographic staple throughout the world of desktop typography and design. Slimbach has captured the beauty and balance of the original Garamond typefaces while creating a typeface family that offers all the advantages of a contemporary digital type family.

The accents are set in Avenir, which was designed by Adrian Frutiger in 1988. The word Avenir means "future" in French and hints that the typeface owes some of its interpretation to the font Futura. But unlike Futura, Avenir is not purely geometric; it has vertical strokes that are thicker than the horizontals, an "o" that is not a perfect circle, and shortened ascenders. These nuances aid in legibility and give Avenir a harmonious and sensible appearance for both texts and headlines.

Text and cover design by Duncan Noel Campbell, University of Regina Press.